PB2002-106364

FTA-MA-26-5010-02-1
DOT-VNTSC-FTA-02-01

U.S. Department
of Transportation

**Federal Transit
Administration**

Drug and Alcohol Testing Results
2000 Annual Report

I0437749

December 2001

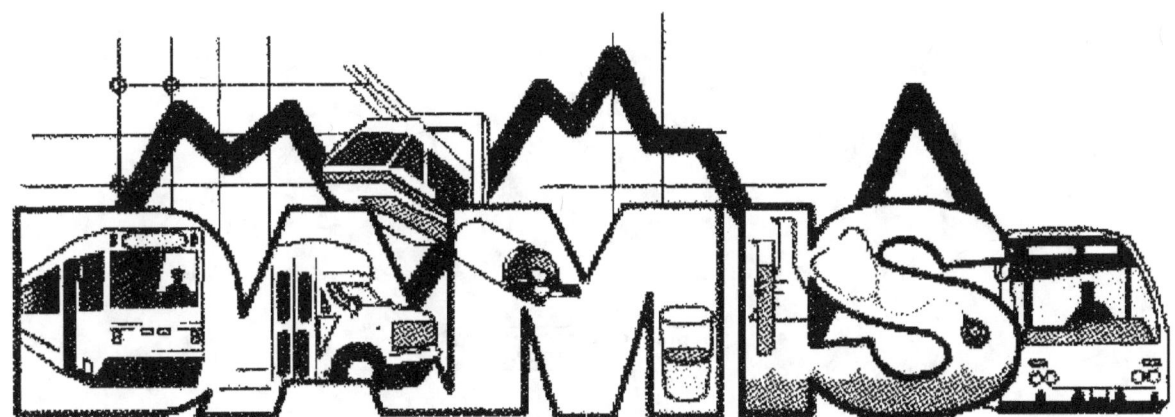

The FTA Drug and Alcohol Management Information System

Office of Safety and Security

Notice

This document is disseminated under the sponsorship of the Department of Transportation in the interest of information exchange. The United States Government assumes no liability for its contents or use thereof.

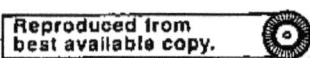

REPORT DOCUMENTATION PAGE

Form Approved
OMB No. 0704-0188

1. AGENCY USE ONLY (Leave blank)	2. REPORT DATE December 2001	3. REPORT TYPE AND DATES COVERED Final Report January 2000–December 2000

4. TITLE AND SUBTITLE
Drug and Alcohol Testing Results 2000 Annual Report

5. FUNDING NUMBERS
TM259/U2139

6. AUTHOR(S)
Richard Anderson,* Brian Baker,** Rene Buchanan, Suzanne Chen, Randy Clarke,* Charity Coleman,* Jessica Paddock,* Michael Redington, and Eve Rutyna*

7. PERFORMING ORGANIZATION NAME(S) AND ADDRESS(ES)
U.S. Department of Transportation
Research and Special Programs Administration
John A. Volpe National Transportation Systems Center
55 Broadway
Cambridge, MA 02142-1093

8. PERFORMING ORGANIZATION REPORT NUMBER
DOT-VNTSC-FTA-02-01

9. SPONSORING/MONITORING AGENCY NAME(S) AND ADDRESS(ES)
U.S. Department of Transportation
Federal Transit Administration
Office of Safety and Security
Washington, DC 20590

10. SPONSORING/MONITORING AGENCY REPORT NUMBER
FTA-MA-26-5010-02-1

11. SUPPLEMENTARY NOTES
* EG&G Technical Services, Inc.   **Cambridge Systematics, Inc.
55 Broadway   150 CambridgePark Drive, Suite 4000
Cambridge, MA 02142-1093   Cambridge, MA 02140

12a. DISTRIBUTION/AVAILABILITY STATEMENT
This document is available to the public through the National Technical Information Service, Springfield, VA 22161

12b. DISTRIBUTION CODE

13. ABSTRACT (Maximum 200 words)

The Drug and Alcohol Testing Results 2000 Annual Report is a compilation and analysis of drug and alcohol testing results reported by transit systems in the United States during 2000. The report covers results for the following drug types: marijuana (THC), cocaine, phencyclidine (PCP), opiates, and amphetamines. The drug test types covered are: pre-employment, random, post-accident, reasonable suspicion, return-to-duty, and follow-up. The report also covers testing results for alcohol for the following test types: random, post-accident, reasonable suspicion, return-to-duty, and follow-up. Now that there are 5 years worth of data, the report has an increased focus on trend analysis.

14. SUBJECT TERMS
alcohol testing, drug testing, FTA-covered employees, random testing, safety sensitive, violation rate

15. NUMBER OF PAGES
96

16. PRICE CODE

17. SECURITY CLASSIFICATION OF REPORT Unclassified	18. SECURITY CLASSIFICATION OF THIS PAGE Unclassified	19. SECURITY CLASSIFICATION OF THIS ABSTRACT Unclassified	20. LIMITATION OF ABSTRACT Unlimited

NSN 7540-01-280-5500

Standard Form 298 (Rev. 2-89)
Prescribed by ANSI Std. 239-18
298-102

PREFACE

This annual report represents the cooperative efforts of many people. Extensive appreciation is extended to the U.S. Department of Transportation's Federal Transit Administration, the Volpe National Transportation Systems Center, and the following individuals who were instrumental in guiding this project and contributing to its success:

Mark A. Snider
Drug and Alcohol Program Manager
Federal Transit Administration

James A. Harrison
Transportation Industry Analyst
Volpe National Transportation Systems Center

Michael R. Redington
Transportation Industry Analyst
Volpe National Transportation Systems Center

METRIC/ENGLISH CONVERSION FACTORS

ENGLISH TO METRIC

LENGTH (APPROXIMATE)

1 inch (in) = 2.5 centimeters (cm)

1 foot (ft) = 30 centimeters (cm)

1 yard (yd) = 0.9 meter (m)

1 mile (mi) = 1.6 kilometers (km)

AREA (APPROXIMATE)

1 square inch (sq in, in²) = 6.5 square centimeters (cm²)

1 square foot (sq ft, ft²) = 0.09 square meter (m²)

1 square yard (sq yd, yd²) = 0.8 square meter (m²)

1 square mile (sq mi, mi²) = 2.6 square kilometers (km²)

1 acre = 0.4 hectare (he) = 4,000 square meters (m²)

MASS - WEIGHT (APPROXIMATE)

1 ounce (oz) = 28 grams (gm)

1 pound (lb) = 0.45 kilogram (kg)

1 short ton = 2,000 pounds (lb) = 0.9 tonne (t)

VOLUME (APPROXIMATE)

1 teaspoon (tsp) = 5 milliliters (ml)

1 tablespoon (tbsp) = 15 milliliters (ml)

1 fluid ounce (fl oz) = 30 milliliters (ml)

1 cup (c) = 0.24 liter (l)

1 pint (pt) = 0.47 liter (l)

1 quart (qt) = 0.96 liter (l)

1 gallon (gal) = 3.8 liters (l)

1 cubic foot (cu ft, ft³) = 0.03 cubic meter (m³)

1 cubic yard (cu yd, yd³) = 0.76 cubic meter (m³)

TEMPERATURE (EXACT)

[(x-32)(5/9)] °F = y °C

METRIC TO ENGLISH

LENGTH (APPROXIMATE)

1 millimeter (mm) = 0.04 inch (in)

1 centimeter (cm) = 0.4 inch (in)

1 meter (m) = 3.3 feet (ft)

1 meter (m) = 1.1 yards (yd)

1 kilometer (km) = 0.6 mile (mi)

AREA (APPROXIMATE)

1 square centimeter (cm²) = 0.16 square inch (sq in, in²)

1 square meter (m²) = 1.2 square yards (sq yd, yd²)

1 square kilometer (km²) = 0.4 square mile (sq mi, mi²)

10,000 square meters (m²) = 1 hectare (ha) = 2.5 acres

MASS - WEIGHT (APPROXIMATE)

1 gram (gm) = 0.036 ounce (oz)

1 kilogram (kg) = 2.2 pounds (lb)

1 tonne (t) = 1,000 kilograms (kg)

= 1.1 short tons

VOLUME (APPROXIMATE)

1 milliliter (ml) = 0.03 fluid ounce (fl oz)

1 liter (l) = 2.1 pints (pt)

1 liter (l) = 1.06 quarts (qt)

1 liter (l) = 0.26 gallon (gal)

1 cubic meter (m³) = 36 cubic feet (cu ft, ft³)

1 cubic meter (m³) = 1.3 cubic yards (cu yd, yd³)

TEMPERATURE (EXACT)

[(9/5) y + 32] °C = x °F

QUICK INCH - CENTIMETER LENGTH CONVERSION

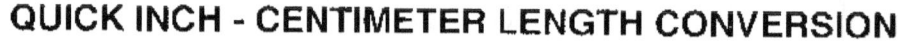
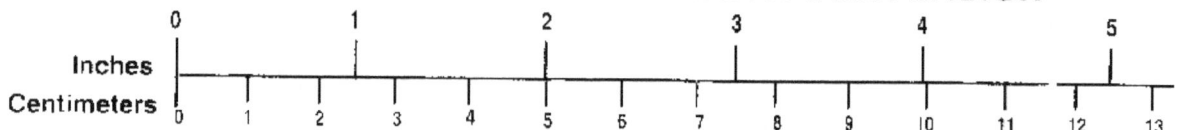

QUICK FAHRENHEIT - CELSIUS TEMPERATURE CONVERSION

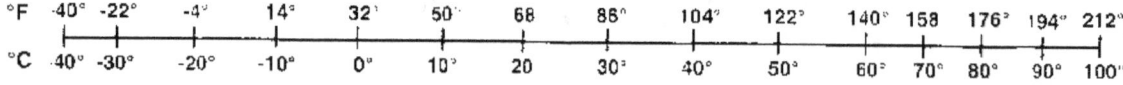

For more exact and or other conversion factors, see NIST Miscellaneous Publication 286. Units of Weights and Measures. Price $2.50 SD Catalog No. C13 10286

Updated 8/17/98

iv

TABLE OF CONTENTS

Section	Page

TABLE OF CONTENTS (cont.)

LIST OF FIGURES

LIST OF FIGURES (cont.)

LIST OF TABLES

LIST OF TABLES (cont.)

EXECUTIVE SUMMARY

INTRODUCTION

This annual report presents the results of mandatory drug and alcohol testing conducted by transit systems and their contractors who receive funds from the Federal Transit Administration (FTA). Under the Omnibus Transportation Employee Testing Act passed by Congress in 1991, the FTA was required to establish regulations for drug and alcohol testing of transit employees performing safety-sensitive functions. These regulations require that each recipient of FTA funds: (1) implement an anti-drug program to deter and detect the use of prohibited drugs, (2) establish a program to prevent the misuse of alcohol, and (3) report the results of its programs to FTA annually. The 2000 Annual Report is the sixth annual report summarizing the reported results of drug and alcohol tests from all such transit systems.

Compliance with FTA's drug and alcohol testing program is a condition of federal assistance. Failure of a recipient to establish and implement a drug and alcohol testing program – either in its own operations or in those of an entity operating on its behalf – may result in the suspension of federal transit funding to the recipient. Because a recipient may not always directly provide mass transit services, the FTA uses the term "operator" or "employer" to describe those who actually provide transit services. The direct recipient of FTA funds, however, is the entity legally responsible to the FTA for compliance.

DISTRIBUTION OF TRANSIT SYSTEMS AND CONTRACTORS

The FTA received drug and alcohol MIS reporting forms for calendar year 2000 from 2,657 individual employers representing 1,700 transit systems and 957 contractors. Of the individual employers, 869 were large operators, 372 were small operators, and 1,416 were rural operators. A total of 1,657 of all employers reported being a member of a consortium. Approximately 74 percent of all employers reported no positive drug test results, and 97 percent of employers reported no alcohol test results ≥ 0.04 percent. The number of contractors who had at least one positive drug test result was 33.8 percent, compared to 21.6 percent of transit systems. The number of contractors who submitted forms with at least one alcohol test result ≥ 0.04 percent was 3.2 percent, compared to 21.6 percent of transit systems.

Employers reported a total of 249,733 employees performing safety-sensitive functions: 78.5 percent of these employees are employed at transit systems and 21.5 percent are employed by contractors. The average transit system employs more than twice as many safety-sensitive employees than the average contractor, 115 to 56. Large operators employ an average of 226 safety-sensitive employees compared to 52 for small operators and 26.4 for rural. The largest number of employees performing safety-sensitive functions are engaged in revenue vehicle operation (70 percent) followed by revenue vehicle and equipment maintenance (18.9 percent). Revenue vehicle control/dispatch, CDL/non-revenue vehicle employees, and armed security personnel combined make-up less 11.0 percent of the overall labor force (7.6 percent, 1.9 percent, and 1.5 percent respectively).

The largest number of contract employees were involved in revenue vehicle operation at 77.2 percent, followed by revenue vehicle and equipment maintenance at 12.9 percent. For rural operators, contractors comprise a relatively small percent of the total number of FTA-covered employees at 19.9 percent; for large operators, contractors comprise a slightly higher total at 20.8 percent. Contractors comprise 31.9 percent of the total number of FTA-covered employees for small contractors.

ELECTRONIC REPORTING

Electronically reporting Drug and Alcohol MIS results became an option for FTA-covered employers in 1998. Electronic software was developed with help and validation capabilities in an effort to lessen the reporting burden. In 2000, 707 employers (27 percent) reported electronically in 2000, versus 568 (22 percent) in 1999.

DRUG TEST RESULTS

The 2000 drug-testing program performed by large, small, and rural FTA-covered employers revealed the following major findings:

- A total of 121,668 specimens were collected for random drug testing: 1,151 of these specimens tested positive for one or more of the five prohibited drugs. Random drug testing accounted for 0.54 percent of the total specimens collected and .32 percent of the total positive specimens.

- The positive random test rate was 1.05 percent industry-wide. Positive test rates were 0.85 percent for transit systems, and 1.85 percent for contractors.

- A total of 226,679 specimens were collected for all six types of drug testing. Of that figure, 3,583 specimens tested positive for one or more of the five prohibited drugs. Transit systems accounted for 72 percent of all drug tests conducted, with contractors accounting for the remaining 28 percent of the total drug tests. The overall percentage (transit systems and contractors combined) of positive drug tests was 1.59 percent.

- Of the six drug test types (pre-employment, random, post-accident, reasonable suspicion, return-to-duty, and follow-up), the highest percent of positive specimens was for reasonable suspicion testing (5.5 percent). Contractors reported positive results at a higher rate than did transit systems in all test types. The lowest percentage of positive specimens was for random testing (0.95 percent).

- Marijuana and cocaine were detected most frequently in the specimens that tested positive for drugs. Of 1,151 random positive specimens, 60.08 percent tested positive for marijuana and 35.56 percent tested positive for cocaine. Marijuana was also detected most frequently in all 10 regions. Forty-five specimens tested positive for multiple drugs; the most common multiple-drug combination was marijuana and cocaine, with 20 positive results.

- There were 240 qualifying accidents that resulted in a positive post-accident drug test (126 from transit systems and 114 from contractors). There was one fatality resulting from these accidents. Marijuana was detected in 50 percent of all positive post-accident drug tests; cocaine was second at 43.3 percent.

ALCOHOL TEST RESULTS

Employers are required to establish and conduct an alcohol misuse prevention program in which employees performing safety-sensitive functions are tested for the misuse of alcohol and supervisors are trained to recognize the signs and symptoms of alcohol misuse. Employees are subject to five types of alcohol tests: random, reasonable suspicion, post-accident, return-to-duty, and follow-up. In addition, employers may not allow safety-sensitive employees to consume alcohol under four specific circumstances: (1) 4 hours before performing a safety-sensitive function; (2) while performing a safety-sensitive function; (3) after a fatal accident, unless the employee has received a post-accident test or 8 hours have elapsed, whichever occurs first; or (4) after a non-fatal accident unless the employee's involvement was completely discounted as a contributing factor to the accident, the employee has been tested, or 8 hours have elapsed.

An employee with an alcohol concentration of 0.02 or greater, but less than 0.04, must be removed from duty for 8 hours or until a retest shows an alcohol concentration of less than 0.02. An employee with an alcohol concentration ≥ 0.04 must be prohibited from performing any safety-sensitive duties, removed from his/her safety-sensitive position, and be evaluated by a substance abuse professional. If the employer has a second-chance policy, the employee must properly complete a course of treatment prescribed by the substance abuse professional, and pass a return-to-duty alcohol test prior to returning to a safety-sensitive position.

The 2000 alcohol-testing program performed by large, small, and rural transit employers revealed the following:

- Of the total 41,002 random alcohol-screening tests conducted, 42 confirmation test results that were ≥ 0.04 were documented (0.10 percent). The percentage of random positive results for transit systems was 0.10 percent, while the percentage of random positive results for contractors was 0.12 percent.

- The FTA alcohol-testing rule includes a definition for the violation rate. The violation rate means the sum of the annual number of results from random alcohol tests conducted that have alcohol concentrations of 0.04 or greater, plus the annual number of refusals to submit to alcohol tests, divided by the sum of the annual number of random alcohol tests, plus the annual number of refusals to submit to a drug test. The violation rate for 2000 for all employers (transit systems and contractors) was 0.15 percent.

- The percent of total alcohol screening results that were ≥ 0.04 for all test types was 0.20 percent industry-wide. The percent for transit systems was 0.18 percent, versus 0.28 percent for contractors.

- Transit systems conducted 80 percent of the 69,005 total screening tests; contractors conducted 20 percent of the total.

- Of the 5 required alcohol test types, the highest percent of test results that were ≥ 0.04 was for reasonable suspicion testing at 7.77 percent. Contractors had nearly double the number of alcohol concentrations at ≥ 0.04 for reasonable suspicion testing than transit systems at 12.02 percent.

- Of the 5 employee categories, the highest percent of test results that were ≥ 0.04 was tied between revenue vehicle control dispatch and CDL/non-revenue vehicle at 0.26 percent. Armed Security Personnel had zero test results ≥ 0.04.

- There were 6 accidents reported that resulted in a post-accident alcohol test result of 0.04 or greater. There were no fatalities resulting from these accidents. Transit systems accounted for all 6 of the post-accident test results ≥ 0.04.

- There were 51 alcohol test refusals: 25 for transit systems and 26 for contractors. Twenty-one refusals were for random tests and 30 were for non-random tests.

- There were 26 reported "other" alcohol violations — 3 of the 4 additional specific circumstances in which employers may not allow their safety-sensitive employees to consume alcohol, as mentioned previously.

TRENDS: 1996 THROUGH 2000

The number of FTA drug and alcohol reporting forms received between 1996 and 2000 increased by 16.18 percent. The greatest gain has been in the number of contractor reports received: reports received from contractors have jumped by 35.40 percent while transit systems have increased by 7.06 percent.

From 1996 to 2000, the number of reported safety-sensitive employees has increased by 12.46 percent for transit systems, and 36.43 percent for contractors. The percent of contracted FTA-covered employees out of the total pool (i.e., including transit systems), increased from 18.44 percent in 1996 to 25.16 percent in 2000.

Overall, the percent of positive random drug test results and the percent of random alcohol test results ≥ 0.04 decreased each year for the 5-year period (see "Totals" column in Tables ES-1 and ES-2).

Table ES-1. 1996 to 2000 Positive Random Drug Test Results

Employer	1996	1997	1998	1999	2000
Transit Systems	1.42%	1.06%	0.93%	0.83%	0.77%
Contractors	1.84%	1.92%	1.69%	1.72%	1.64%
Totals	1.50%	1.21%	1.07%	1.00%	0.95%

Table ES-2. 1996 to 2000 Random Alcohol Test Results ≥ 0.04

Employer	1996	1997	1998	1999	2000
Transit Systems	0.17%	0.15%	0.13%	0.10%	0.10%
Contractors	0.11%	0.09%	0.14%	0.05%	0.12%
Totals	0.16%	0.14%	0.13%	0.09%	0.10%

As with random testing, the percent of positive drug test results decreased overall each year for the 5-year period from 1996 to 2000. Transit systems showed a significant decrease in total positive drug tests, whereas the percent of total positive drug tests for contractors showed no trend. See Table ES-3 below for the percentages. See Table ES-4 for the percent of total alcohol test results ≥ 0.04 for both transit systems and contractors.

Table ES-3. 1996 to 2000 Percent of Positive Drug Test Results

Employer	1996	1997	1998	1999	2000
Transit Systems	1.75%	1.41%	1.28%	1.20%	1.12%
Contractors	2.75%	3.01%	2.87%	2.66%	2.78%
Totals	2.00%	1.77%	1.67%	1.59%	1.58%

Table ES-4. 1996 to 2000 Percent of Alcohol Test Results ≥ 0.04

Employer	1996	1997	1998	1999	2000
Transit Systems	0.26%	0.23%	0.24%	0.18%	0.18%
Contractors	0.27%	0.28%	0.56%	0.33%	0.28%
Totals	0.26%	0.24%	0.29%	0.21%	0.20%

See Table ES-5 and ES-6 for positive drug and alcohol tests ≥ 0.04 for all 5 employee category types over the last 5 years.

Table ES-5. 1996 to 2000 Percent of Positive Drug Test Results/ Employee Category

Employer	1996	1997	1998	1999	2000
Revenue Vehicle Operation	2.06%	1.87%	1.79%	1.70%	1.72%
Revenue Veh. And Equip. Maint.	1.95%	1.69%	1.45%	1.46%	1.32%
Revenue Veh. Control/Disp.	1.20%	0.91%	0.85%	0.97%	0.80%
CDL/Non-Revenue Vehicle	2.55%	2.05%	2.06%	1.02%	1.13%
Armed Security Personnel	0.73%	0.28%	0.60%	0.53%	0.41%
Totals	2.00%	1.77%	1.67%	1.59%	1.58%

Table ES-6. 1996 to 2000 Alcohol Test Results ≥ 0.04/ Employee Category

Employer	1996	1997	1998	1999	2000
Revenue Vehicle Operation	0.23%	0.20%	0.26%	0.17%	0.21%
Revenue Veh. And Equip. Maint.	0.33%	0.34%	0.39%	0.33%	0.19%
Revenue Veh. Control/Disp.	0.20%	0.30%	0.47%	0.30%	0.26%
CDL/Non-Revenue Vehicle	0.61%	0.48%	0.42%	0.26%	0.26%
Armed Security Personnel	0.06%	0.06%	0.00%	0.00%	0.00%
Totals	0.26%	0.24%	0.29%	0.21%	0.20%

1. INTRODUCTION

This annual report presents the results of mandatory drug and alcohol testing conducted by transit systems that receive funds from the Federal Transit Administration (FTA). Under the Omnibus Transportation Employee Testing Act passed by Congress in 1991, the FTA was required to establish regulations for drug and alcohol testing of transit employees who perform safety-sensitive functions. The purpose of requiring transit agencies to implement drug and alcohol programs is to achieve a drug- and alcohol-free work force in the interest of the health and safety of transit employees and the traveling public. This report covers the testing results from the calendar year 2000, as well as trend analysis dating back to the program's inception.

The FTA regulations require that recipients of specific FTA funds implement an anti-drug program to deter and detect the use of prohibited drugs by transit employees, and to establish a program to prevent prohibited alcohol use. Covered under these regulations are employees of transit systems who receive grant funds, and employees of contractors to those transit systems. Large operators (i.e., those providing transit services in urbanized areas of 200,000 or more in population) were required to begin their drug and alcohol testing programs for calendar year 1995. Small operators (i.e., those providing transit services in areas of less than 200,000) were required to begin their drug and alcohol testing programs for calendar year 1996.

1.1 Who Must Report

Transit systems that receive funding from the FTA sources listed in Figure 1-1 are required to have drug and alcohol testing programs. Under FTA regulations, all recipients must implement the required drug and alcohol testing programs and must report the results of their programs to the FTA annually. The results must be submitted to the FTA on specific Management Information System (MIS) forms or data diskettes. For the 2000 reporting year, a sample of transit agencies reported over the Internet, testing this next reporting option, which will be available for 2001 reporting. Recipients of 5310 funds only are not required to comply with FTA drug and alcohol testing requirements, unless they provide contract services to recipients receiving Section 5307, 5309, and 5311 funds. In those instances, they must report as contractors.

Section 5307 (Section 9). Formula Program

Section 5309 (Section 3). Capital Program

Section 5310 (Section 16). Elderly and Disabled Program

Section 5311 (Section 18). Non-urbanized Area Program

Figure 1-1. FTA Federal Funding Sources

Section 5307 refers to block grants for capital projects and to finance the planning, improvement, and operating costs of equipment, facilities, and associated capital maintenance items for use in mass transportation. Section 5309 refers to discretionary grants and loans for capital projects, new and existing fixed guideway systems, an efficient mass transportation system coordinated with other transportation systems, the introduction of new technologies, the enhancement of urban economic development or the incorporation of private investment, and mass transportation projects to meet the needs of the elderly and individuals with disabilities. Section 5310 refers to grants and loans for the special needs of the elderly and individuals with disabilities. Section 5311 refers to financial assistance for non-urbanized areas.

Some recipients provide mass transit services directly. Others rely on additional public or private entities to provide services in whole or in part. In these cases, the direct recipient of FTA funds is legally responsible for assuring that any entity operating on its behalf is in compliance with FTA testing rules.

Transit systems that receive funding directly from the FTA must certify annually that they are in compliance with the drug and alcohol testing regulations. States must certify regulatory compliance on behalf of the transit systems that receive FTA funding through a state agency.

Failure of a recipient to establish and implement a drug and alcohol testing program, either in its own operations or in those of an entity operating on its behalf, may result in the suspension of federal transit funding to the recipient. Because a recipient may not always provide transit services directly, the FTA uses the term "operator" or "employer" to describe those who actually provide transit services and who therefore, must implement the FTA requirements.

1.2   Employees Who Must be Tested

Under the FTA's drug and alcohol testing regulations, employees and supervisors who perform any of the following functions are considered safety-sensitive employees:

1. Operate a revenue service vehicle, including when not in revenue service (includes employees who operate a passenger vehicle, whether or not a fare is collected);

2. Maintain revenue service vehicles or equipment used in revenue service (except 5311 recipients' contractors);

3. Dispatch or control revenue service vehicles;

4. Operate a non-revenue service vehicle (e.g., ancillary vehicle), which requires a Commercial Drivers License (CDL), and is not already covered by another employee category; and/or

5. Provide security and carry a firearm.

Maintenance contractors (except for 5311 recipients' contractors) who perform routine, ongoing repair or maintenance work for FTA recipients and subrecipients must comply with the regulations if their employees perform any of the identified safety-sensitive functions. In addition, supervisors who perform, or could be called upon to perform, any of the safety-sensitive functions are also included.

1.3   Types of Tests

Employees who perform safety-sensitive functions are subject to six different types of tests:

1) **Pre-employment testing** for drugs is performed on each prospective employee, including individuals who are being transferred into safety-sensitive positions, or who are returning following an absence that resulted in being removed from the random pool. Employees may not be hired unless they have a verified negative drug test result. (This is no longer applicable for alcohol — the FTA suspended required pre-employment testing for alcohol on May 10, 1995, as a result of a U.S. Court of Appeals decision.)

2) **Random testing** must be unannounced and unpredictable. The tests must be based on a scientifically valid random-number selection method. All safety-sensitive employees must have an equal chance of being selected for testing each time a selection is made. They must also be included in the selection pool, and must remain in the pool after being tested. For 2000, the number of random tests conducted must equal at least 50 percent (for drugs) and 10 percent (for alcohol) of the average number of safety-sensitive employees in the random pool at the time of the random draws. Transit systems have the option of joining a consortium; an entity that arranges testing services and that acts on behalf of the employers. If a transit system joins a consortium for random testing, the testing rate applies to the total number of safety-sensitive employees within the random testing pool of the consortium. As a result, some individual transit operators may not appear to meet the random testing requirement.

3) **Post-accident testing** is required for accidents where there is loss of human life. For non-fatal accidents that meet FTA-defined conditions, testing is required unless the covered employee's performance can be completely discounted as a causative or contributing factor. When an accident occurs, safety-sensitive employees operating the vehicle must be tested, as well as any other safety-sensitive personnel not in the vehicle whose performance could have contributed to the accident. Tests must be administered as soon as possible, but no later than 8 hours after the accident for alcohol, and 32 hours post-accident for drugs.

4) **Reasonable suspicion testing** is conducted when an employer suspects that an employee has used a prohibited drug or has misused alcohol as defined in the regulations. Reasonable suspicion determinations are made by trained supervisors and must be based on specific, contemporaneous, articulated observations concerning the appearance, behavior, speech, or body odor of the safety-sensitive employee.

5) **Return-to-duty testing** occurs when an employer's policy statement permits an employee who violated the regulations (i.e., tested positive for drugs, had an alcohol result of ≥ 0.04, refused to submit to a test) to return to duty to perform a safety-sensitive function after completion of rehabilitation. The employee must, however, be evaluated by a Substance Abuse Professional (SAP) and pass a return-to-duty test prior to performing a safety-sensitive function.

6) **Follow-up testing** occurs after an employee has returned to duty following a positive drug or alcohol test. The employee is subject to unannounced follow-up testing for at least 12, but no

more than 60 months as recommended by the SAP. Follow-up testing is separate from, and in addition to, random testing.

1.4   Drug Testing Program Overview

Transit systems must establish an anti-drug program that focuses on testing safety-sensitive employees and training for supervisors. FTA regulations specify that safety-sensitive employees may not use any of the 5 following prohibited substances (or their metabolites): marijuana; cocaine; opiates (e.g., heroin, morphine, codeine); amphetamines (e.g., racemic, amphetamine, extroamphetamine, and methamphetamine); or phencyclidine (PCP). Testing for any other drugs must be performed separately from the FTA test.

If an FTA-covered employee has a verified positive drug test result, the employee must be removed from their safety-sensitive position, be informed of the available educational and treatment programs, and be referred to a SAP. To return to a safety-sensitive position, the employee must complete a course of treatment prescribed by the SAP and take a return-to-duty drug test with a verified negative result.

1.5   Alcohol Testing Program Overview

Transit systems are required to establish and conduct an alcohol misuse prevention program in which employees performing safety-sensitive functions are tested for alcohol misuse. In addition, supervisors must receive specific training to recognize the signs and symptoms of possible alcohol misuse. There are four specific circumstances under which an employee is prohibited from consuming alcohol:

1. Four hours before performing a safety-sensitive function;

2. While performing a safety-sensitive function;

3. After a fatal accident, unless a post-accident test has been administered, or 8 hours have elapsed (whichever occurs first); and/or

4. After a non-fatal accident, unless the employee's involvement can be completely discounted as a contributing factor to the accident, the employee has been tested, or 8 hours has elapsed.

An employee with an alcohol concentration of 0.02 or greater but less than 0.04 for a confirmation test must be removed from duty for at least 8 hours or until a re-test conducted by the employer shows an alcohol concentration of less than 0.02. If an employer elects to remove the employee from duty for 8 hours, the employer is not required to administer an alcohol test before the employee resumes performing a safety-sensitive function, unless the employee exhibits signs of alcohol misuse upon returning to work.

A safety-sensitive employee with an alcohol concentration of ≥ 0.04 must be prohibited from performing any safety-sensitive functions, removed from his or her safety-sensitive position, and be referred to a SAP.

1.6 Drug and Alcohol MIS Data Quality and Validation

The Drug and Alcohol MIS data submitted to the FTA by transit operators and their contractors are subjected to extensive analysis and validation, both manual and automated. The process entails detailed examination of each MIS report, identification of errors or questionable entries, and the resolution of these problems in conjunction with the reporting agencies.

Despite extensive efforts, it should be noted that data validation primarily encompasses a review of the consistency and reasonableness of the reported data. Errors of significant magnitude have been detected and corrected, but some statistically minor errors may remain.

1.7 Availability of Drug and Alcohol MIS Documentation

Copies of reporting guidance and MIS reporting forms and diskettes are available from the Drug and Alcohol MIS Project Office at (617) 494-6336. The FTA Safety and Security Clearinghouse can be reached at (617) 494-2108 for additional copies of this report, as well as previously published annual reports. Other technical assistance materials including the *Implementation Guidelines for Drug and Alcohol Regulations in Mass Transit,* may be acquired from the FTA's Office of Safety & Security at (202) 366-2896. Further information can also be found on the Office of Safety and Security's Web site at the following address: http://transit-safety.volpe.dot.gov/damis.

1.8 Organization of this Report

This report contains five chapters and two appendices. Chapter 2 provides general information on the reporting process, including how many employers reported testing results to the FTA. Chapters 3 and 4 present drug and alcohol testing results, respectively. Chapter 5 presents a trend analysis of testing results from 1996 through 2000. A glossary of terms used throughout this report comprises Appendix A, and Appendix B provides a list of FTA regions.

Last year, an additional size category (rural) was introduced and another size category (small) was, therefore, redefined. "Large" systems are located in urbanized areas of 200,000 or more in population. "Small" systems are located in urbanized areas of less than 200,000, but greater than or equal to 50,000. "Rural" systems are located in areas of less than 50,000 in population.

2. GENERAL INFORMATION ON DRUG AND ALCOHOL FORMS

This chapter graphically presents the data submitted on the 2000 FTA Drug and Alcohol MIS forms. Among the data presented are the number of paper MIS Data Collection forms versus data diskettes* received, and the number of forms received by employer size and region. Also shown are the number of FTA-covered employees by employee category, break outs for transit systems and contractors, and the percent of FTA-covered employees by employer size.

SUMMARY FINDINGS FOR 2000 REPORTING:

- A total of 2,657 MIS Data Collection forms were collected from transit systems and contractors combined, of which 1,950 were in paper form while 707 were reported using the reporting software and submitted on data disk.

- A total of 869 forms were received from large systems, 372 from small systems, and 1,416 from rural systems (transit systems and contractors combined).

- Region 4 had the largest number of employers reporting Drug and Alcohol testing results.

- Region 2 had the highest number of FTA-covered employees, including both transit systems and contractors, while Region 8 had the lowest number.

---

*Beginning in 1998, reporters had the option to report on either paper forms or by using the electronic reporting system and submitting results on a data disk.

2.1 Distribution of Transit Systems and Contractors

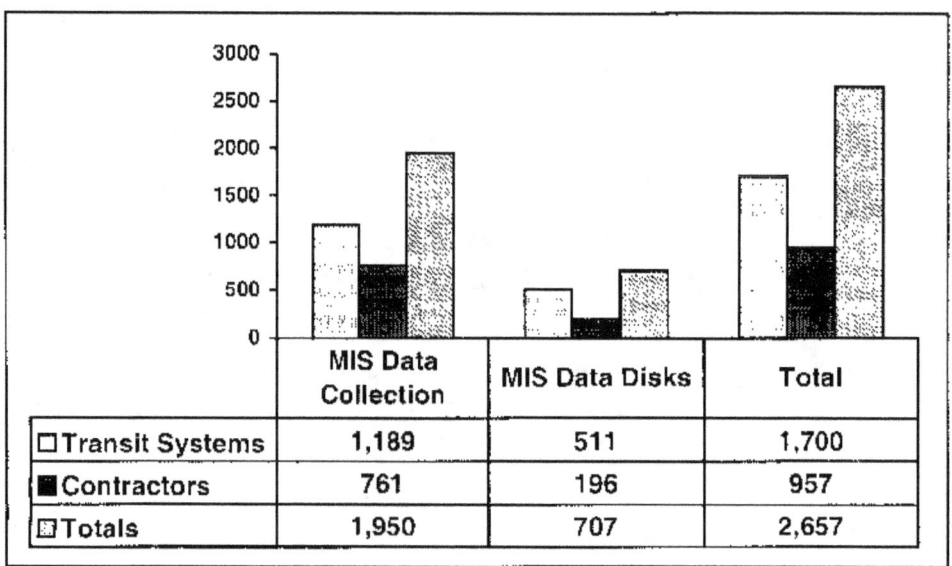

	MIS Data Collection	MIS Data Disks	Total
☐ Transit Systems	1,189	511	1,700
■ Contractors	761	196	957
☐ Totals	1,950	707	2,657

Figure 2-1. Number of Drug and Alcohol Forms Received

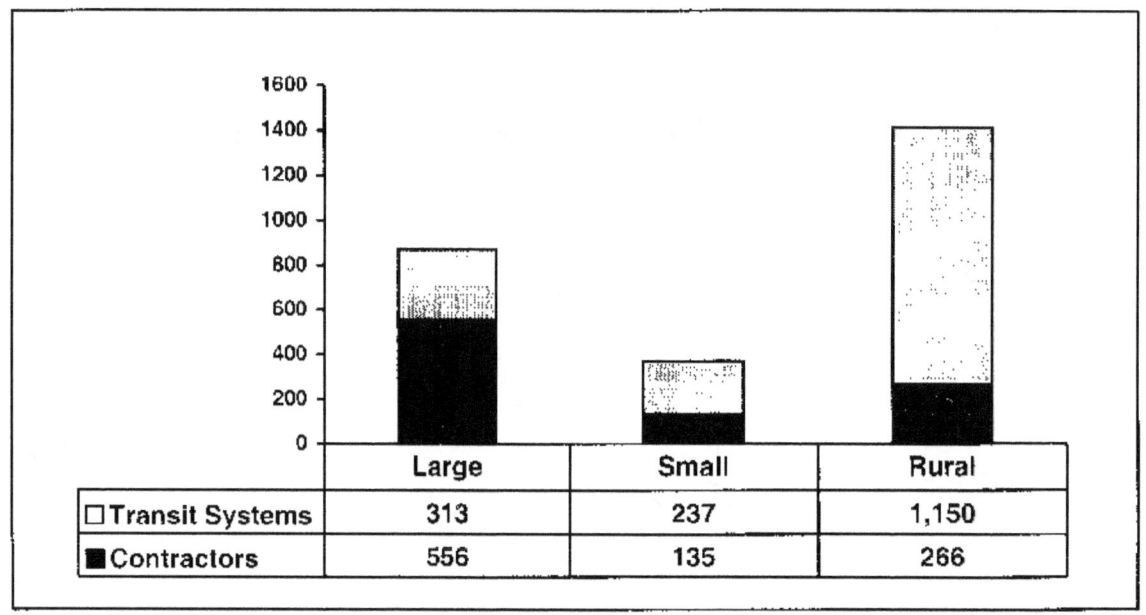

	Large	Small	Rural
☐ Transit Systems	313	237	1,150
■ Contractors	556	135	266

Figure 2-2. Drug and Alcohol Forms Received by Employer Size

2.2 Drug and Alcohol Forms Received by Region

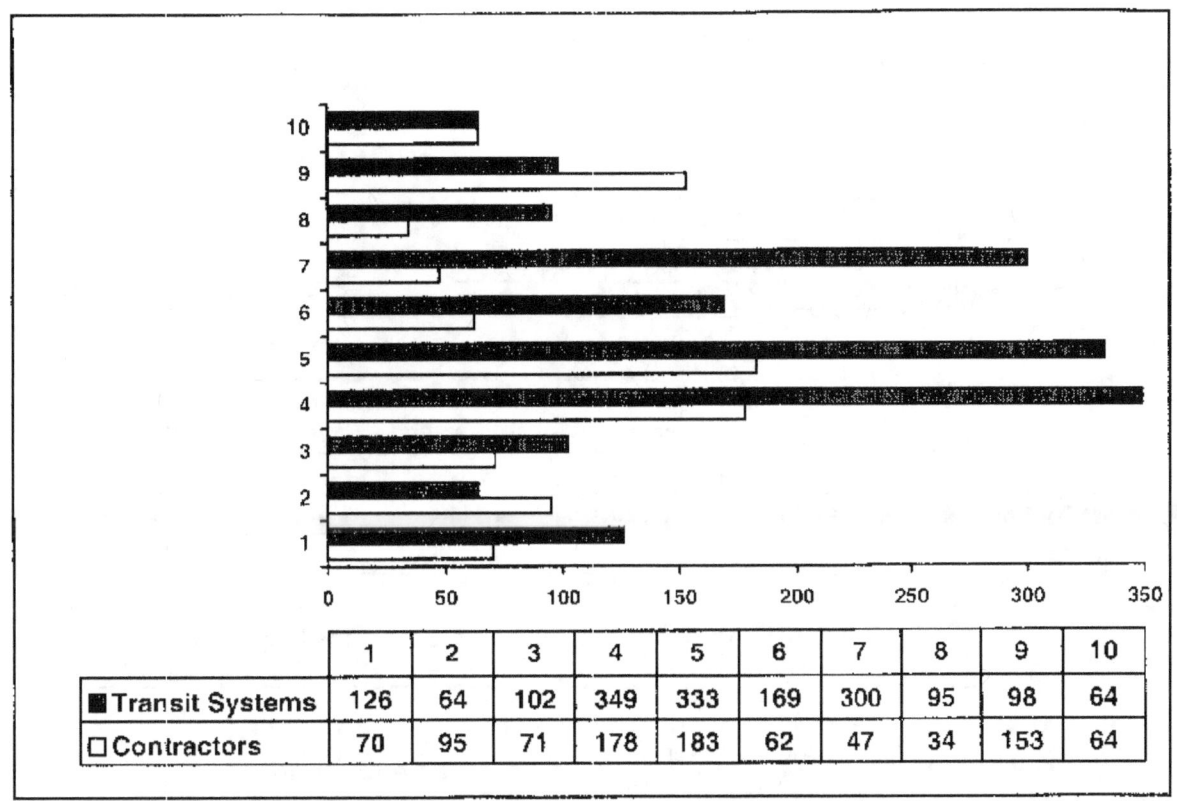

	1	2	3	4	5	6	7	8	9	10
■ Transit Systems	126	64	102	349	333	169	300	95	98	64
□ Contractors	70	95	71	178	183	62	47	34	153	64

Figure 2-3. Number of FTA Drug and Alcohol Forms Received by Region

2.3 FTA-Covered Employees

Following are a variety of break outs for FTA-covered employees: by employee category, by transit system versus contractor, percent of employees for large, small, and rural employers, and finally by region.

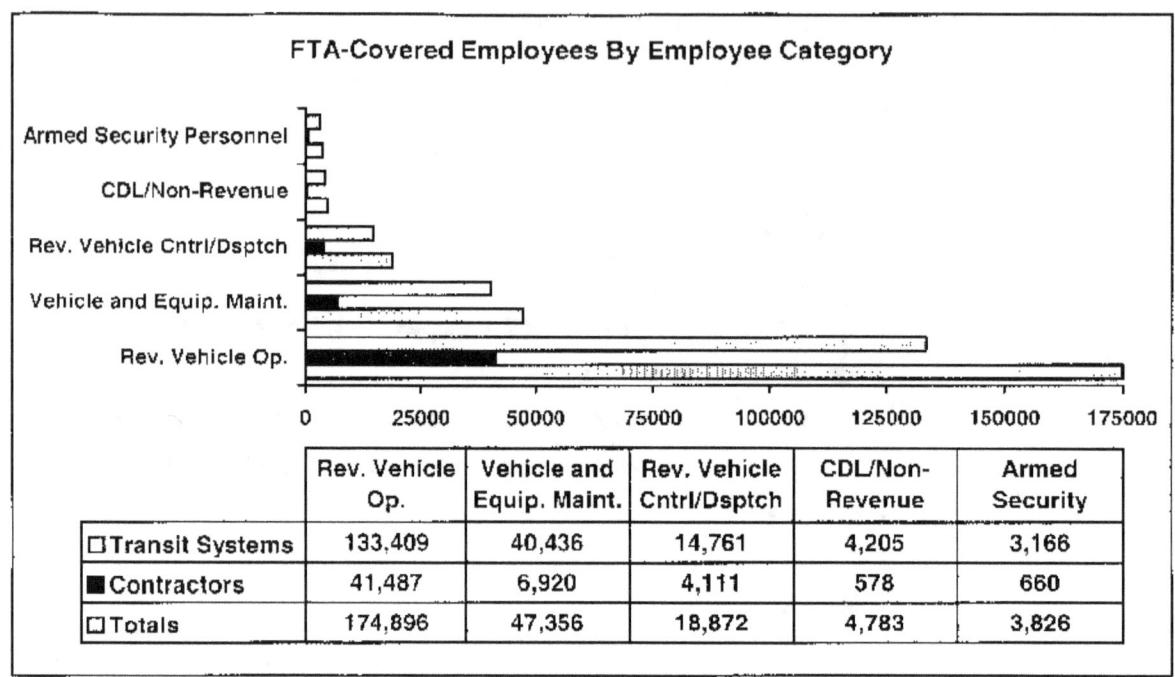

FTA-Covered Employees By Employee Category

	Rev. Vehicle Op.	Vehicle and Equip. Maint.	Rev. Vehicle Cntrl/Dsptch	CDL/Non-Revenue	Armed Security
☐ Transit Systems	133,409	40,436	14,761	4,205	3,166
■ Contractors	41,487	6,920	4,111	578	660
☐ Totals	174,896	47,356	18,872	4,783	3,826

Figure 2-4. Number of FTA-Covered Employees by Employee Category

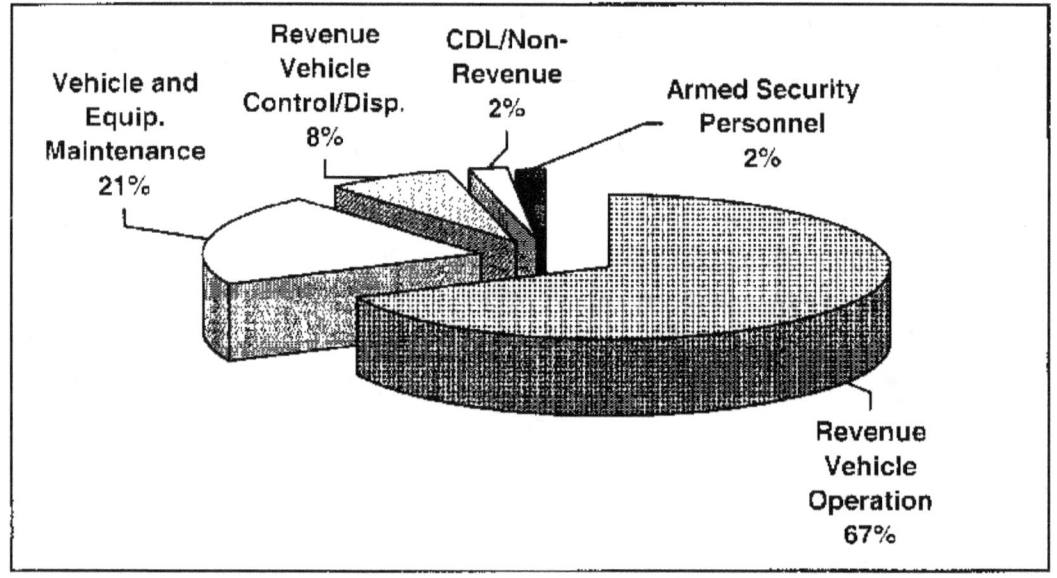

Figure 2-5. Percent of FTA-Covered Employees in Each Employee Category-Transit System

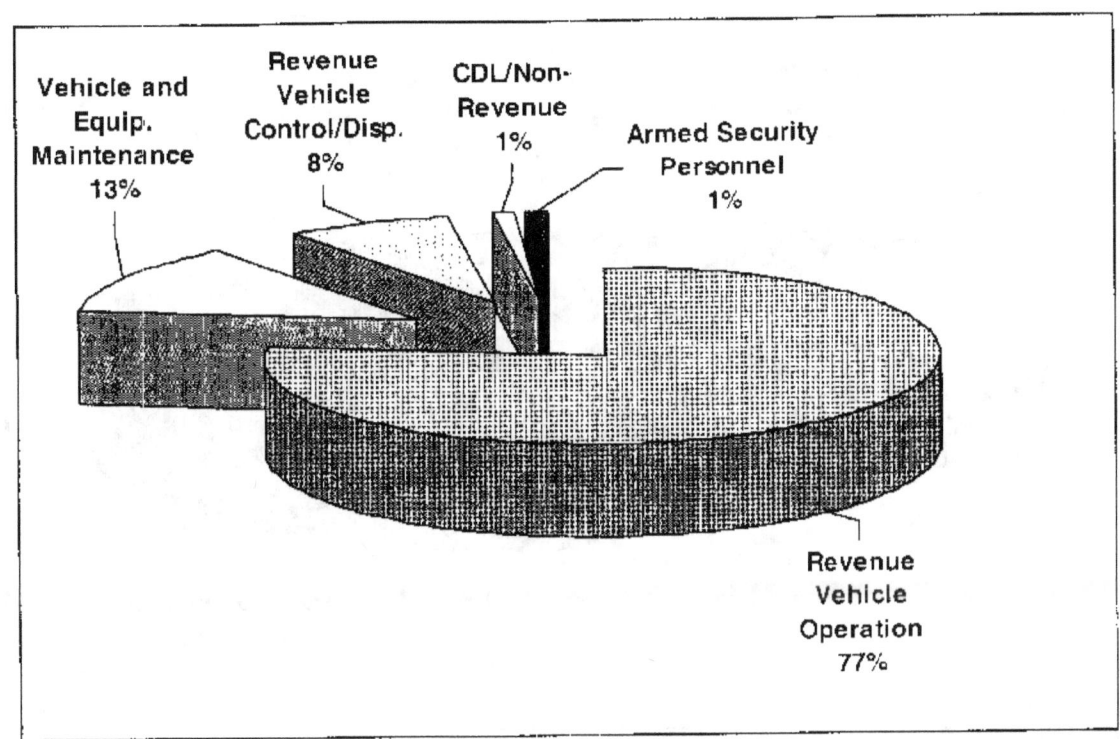

Figure 2-6. Percent of FTA-Covered Employees in Each Employee Category-Contractors

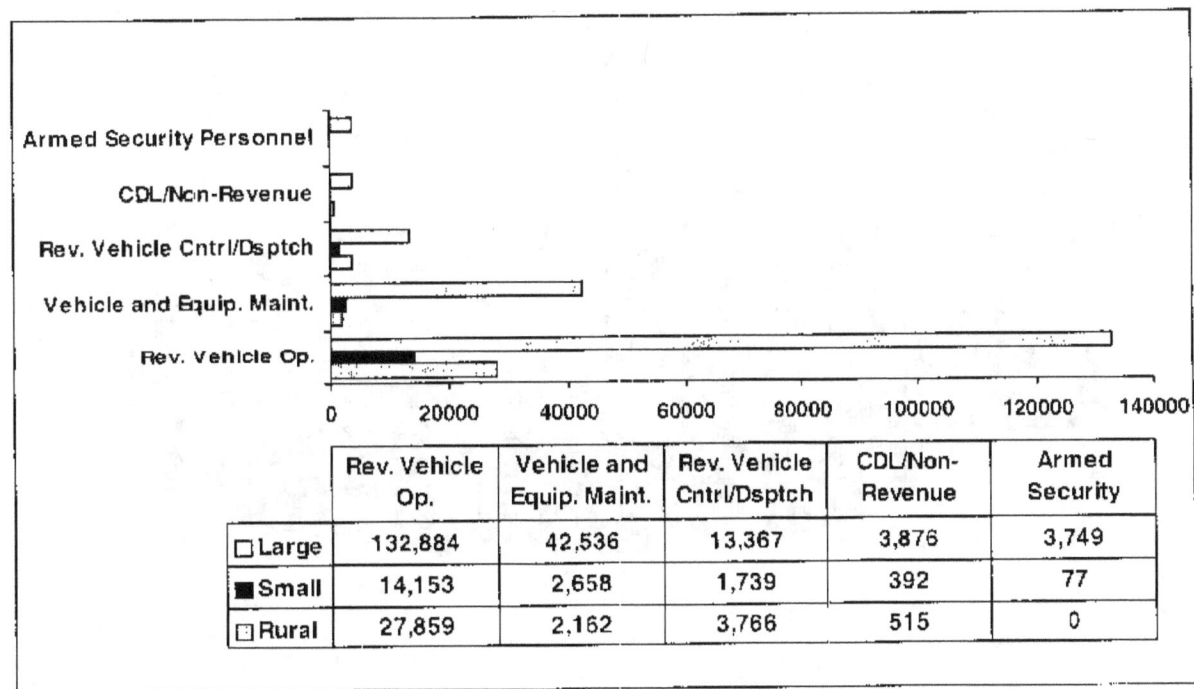

	Rev. Vehicle Op.	Vehicle and Equip. Maint.	Rev. Vehicle Cntrl/Dsptch	CDL/Non-Revenue	Armed Security
☐ Large	132,884	42,536	13,367	3,876	3,749
■ Small	14,153	2,658	1,739	392	77
☐ Rural	27,859	2,162	3,766	515	0

Figure 2-7. Number of FTA-Covered Employees by Employee Category–Large, Small, and Rural Systems

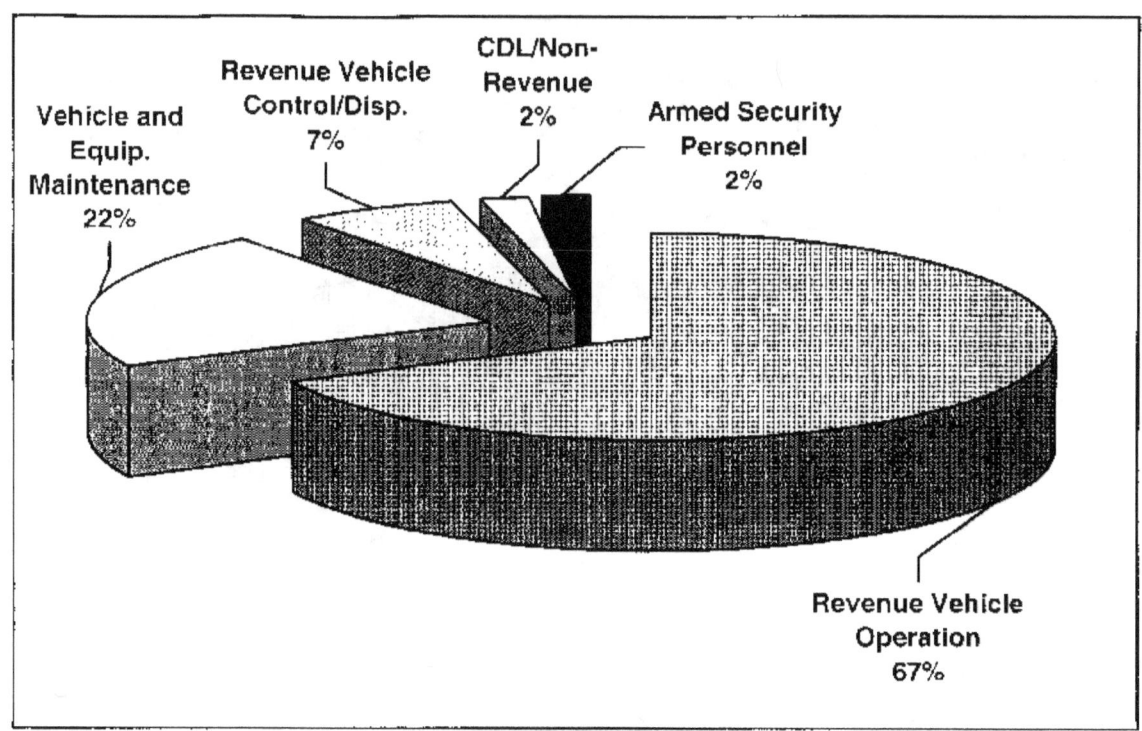

Figure 2-8. Percent of All FTA-Covered Employees for Large Operators

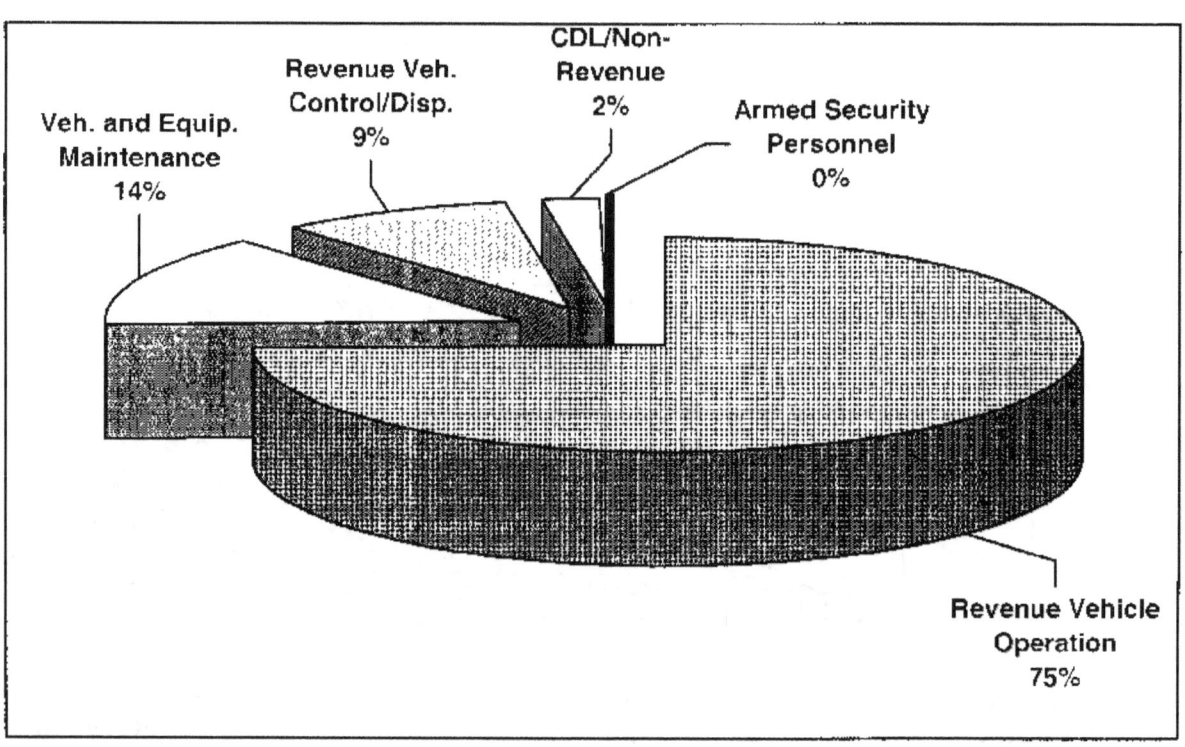

Figure 2-9. Percent of All FTA-Covered Employees for Small Operators

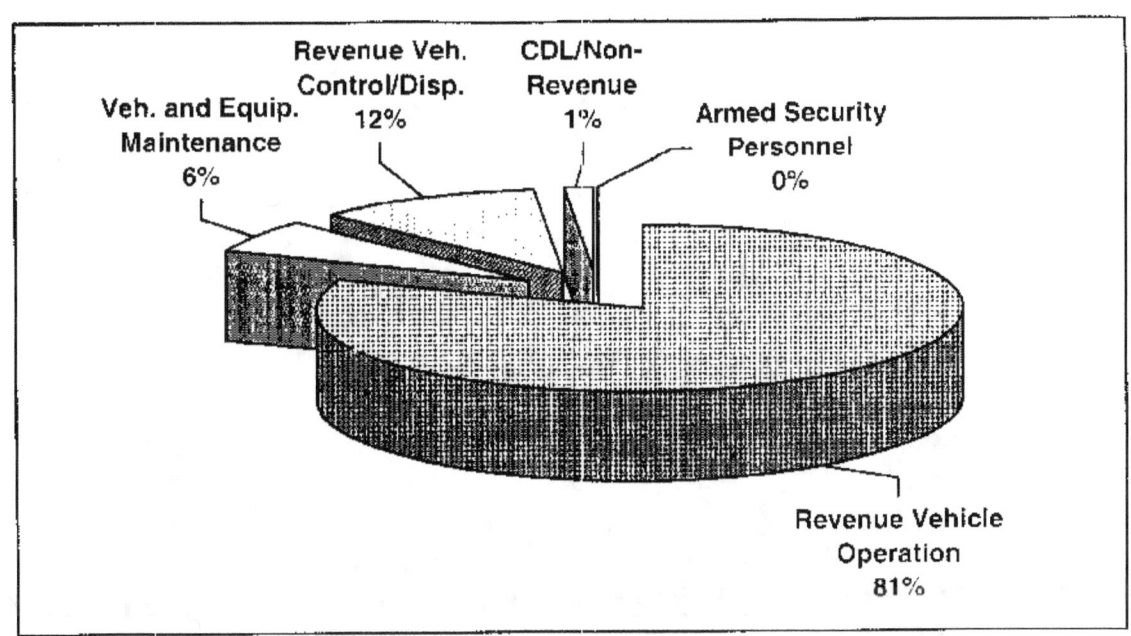

Figure 2-10. Percent of All FTA-Covered Employees Reporting for Rural Operators

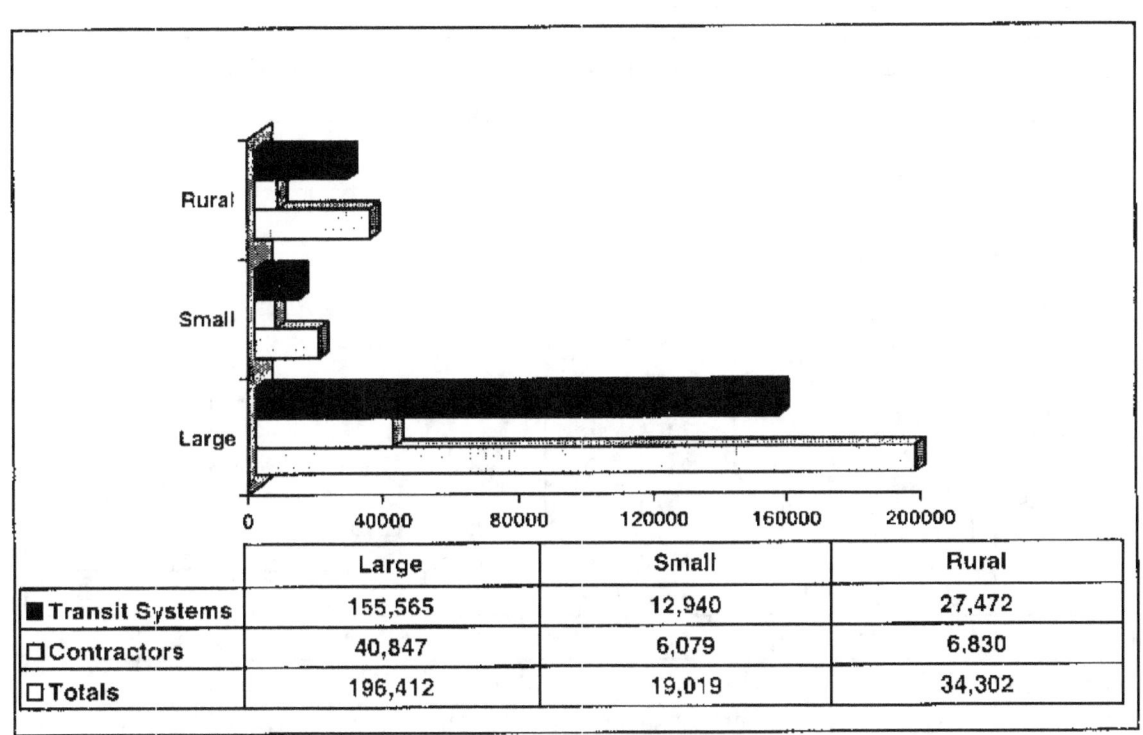

	Large	Small	Rural
■Transit Systems	155,565	12,940	27,472
□Contractors	40,847	6,079	6,830
□Totals	196,412	19,019	34,302

Figure 2-11. Number of FTA-Covered Employees by Employer Size

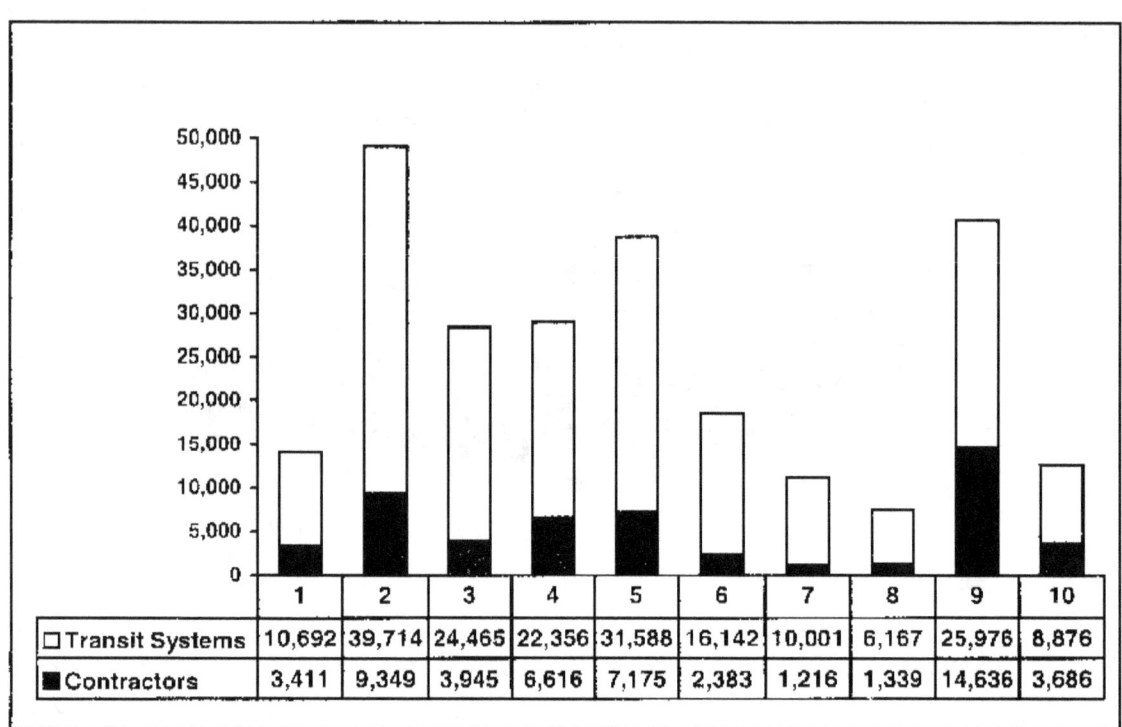

Figure 2-12. Number of FTA-Covered Employees by Region

	1	2	3	4	5	6	7	8	9	10
☐ Transit Systems	10,692	39,714	24,465	22,356	31,588	16,142	10,001	6,167	25,976	8,876
■ Contractors	3,411	9,349	3,945	6,616	7,175	2,383	1,216	1,339	14,636	3,686

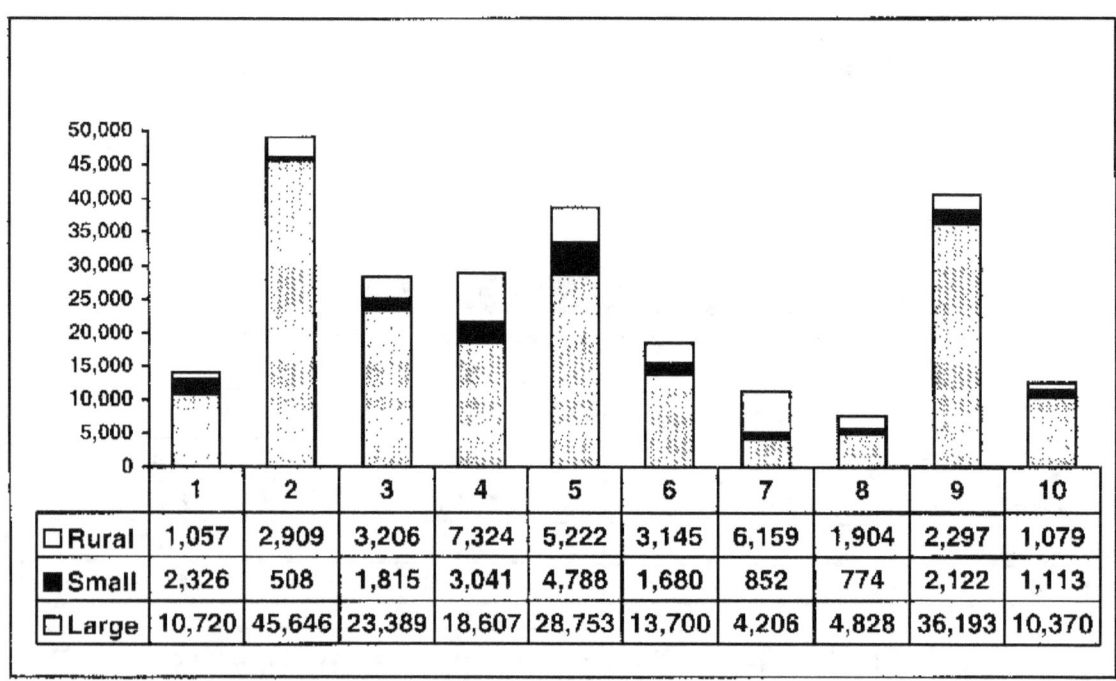

Figure 2-13. FTA-Covered Employees by Region/Size

	1	2	3	4	5	6	7	8	9	10
☐ Rural	1,057	2,909	3,206	7,324	5,222	3,145	6,159	1,904	2,297	1,079
■ Small	2,326	508	1,815	3,041	4,788	1,680	852	774	2,122	1,113
☐ Large	10,720	45,646	23,389	18,607	28,753	13,700	4,206	4,828	36,193	10,370

2.4   Federal Funds

As mentioned in Chapter 1, transit systems are required to report the sources of FTA funds they receive (that is, Sections 5309, 5307, 5310, and 5311). Some of the transit systems receive funding under multiple sections.

The following charts depict the percentage of FTA funding recipients who receive specific funding, and transit systems receiving FTA funds by funding source, as well as by FTA region.

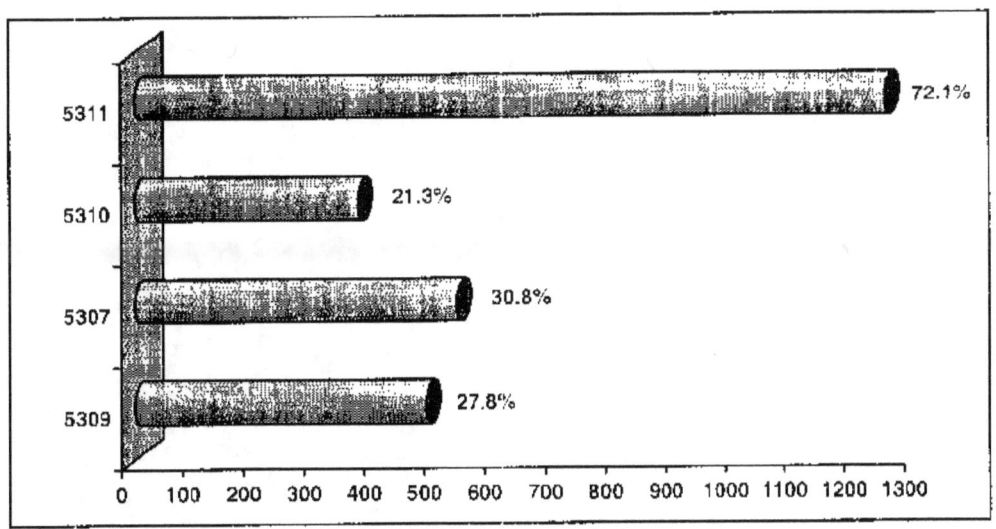

Figure 2-14. Percentage of FTA Funding Recipients Who Receive Specific Funding

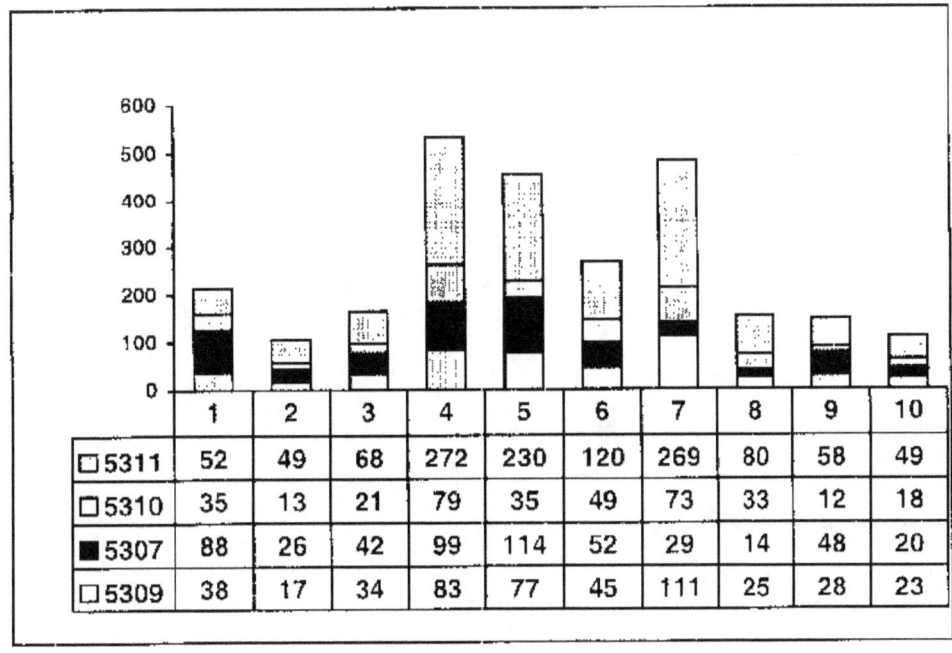

	1	2	3	4	5	6	7	8	9	10
☐ 5311	52	49	68	272	230	120	269	80	58	49
☐ 5310	35	13	21	79	35	49	73	33	12	18
■ 5307	88	26	42	99	114	52	29	14	48	20
☐ 5309	38	17	34	83	77	45	111	25	28	23

Figure 2-15. Number of Transit Systems that Received Federal Funds by Source of Funding and by FTA Region

3. DRUG TEST RESULTS

Chapter 3 provides background information for drug testing results and summarizes drug test results for FTA-funded transit systems and contractors throughout the Administration's regions for 2000. The chapter explains and quantifies the results of testing safety-sensitive employees for prohibited drugs such as marijuana, cocaine, PCP, opiates, and amphetamines.

Six types of tests are administered: pre-employment, random, post-accident, reasonable suspicion, return-to-duty, and follow-up. Of the 226,679 urine specimen collected, 3,583 or 1.59 percent generated verified positive results. To better understand the employers' testing results, the following determinants are charted and graphed for further analysis:

- transit systems versus contractors
- large systems versus small or rural systems
- regional comparisons
- employee categories
- drug type comparisons
- test type comparisons

The results of random drug testing provide the best indication of the overall level of drug usage among FTA-covered transit employees.

SUMMARY OF DRUG TEST RESULTS:

- 1.59% of all specimens collected resulted in a verified positive result.

- The positive rate for random drug tests was 1.04%.

- The percent of random drug test positives was 0.95%.

- Regions 5, 8, and 9 have the highest percentage of verified positive random drug tests at 1.23%, 1.63%, and 1.33%, respectively.

- Regions 6, 8, and 9 have the highest percentage of verified positive drug tests at 2.00%, 2.43%, and 2.20%, respectively.

- Of the total positive results for drug type, THC was present in 58.62% of the specimens collected.

- THC/Cocaine represents 44.4% of multiple drug combinations.

3.1   Positive Drug Rates for 2000

Table 3-1 shows the positive rate results of transit systems and contractors. Table 3-2 illustrates the random drug test results of transit systems and contractors. The positive rate is 1.05%; 0.95% of all random specimens collected resulted in a verified positive result. Positive rate means the sum of the annual number of positive results for random drug tests conducted, plus the annual number of refusals to submit to a random drug test, divided by the sum of the annual number of random drug tests conducted, plus the annual number of refusals to submit to a random drug test.

Random Drug Positives + Random Refusals
_____

Random Drug Tests + Random Refusals

Table 3-3 demonstrates a more in-depth break out of the operator size of the transit systems and contractors based upon the test results. The population that surrounds the transit organization determines the size of operation for each agency. Large, small, and rural organizations are categorized by a population of 200,000 or more, 200,000-50,000, and less than 50,000, respectively.

Table 3-1. 2000 Positive Rate

Employer Type	Number of Specimens	Number Positive	Number of Random Refusals	Positive Rate
Transit Systems	97,185	749	73	0.85%
Contractors	24,483	402	53	1.85%
Totals	121,668	1,151	126	1.05%

Table 3-2. 2000 Random Drug Test Results

Employer Type	Number of Specimens	Number Positive	Percent Positive
Transit Systems	97,185	749	.77%
Contractors	24,483	402	1.64%
Totals	121,668	1,151	.95%

Table 3-3. Random Drug Test Results by Operator Size

Operator Size	Number of Specimens	Number Positive	Percent Positive
Large	96,847	920	.95%
Small	8,963	115	1.28%
Rural	15,858	116	.73%
Totals	121,668	1,151	.95%

3.2 Drug Test Results by FTA Region

Figures 3-1 and 3-2 demonstrate the positive results for random and overall tests, respectively. As shown in Figure 3-1, of the ten FTA regions, Regions 8 and 9 had the highest percent of random specimens testing positive for one or more drugs. Figure 3-2 shows the percentage of drug positives in each category by FTA region. Regions 8 and 9 had the highest percent of drug positives overall.

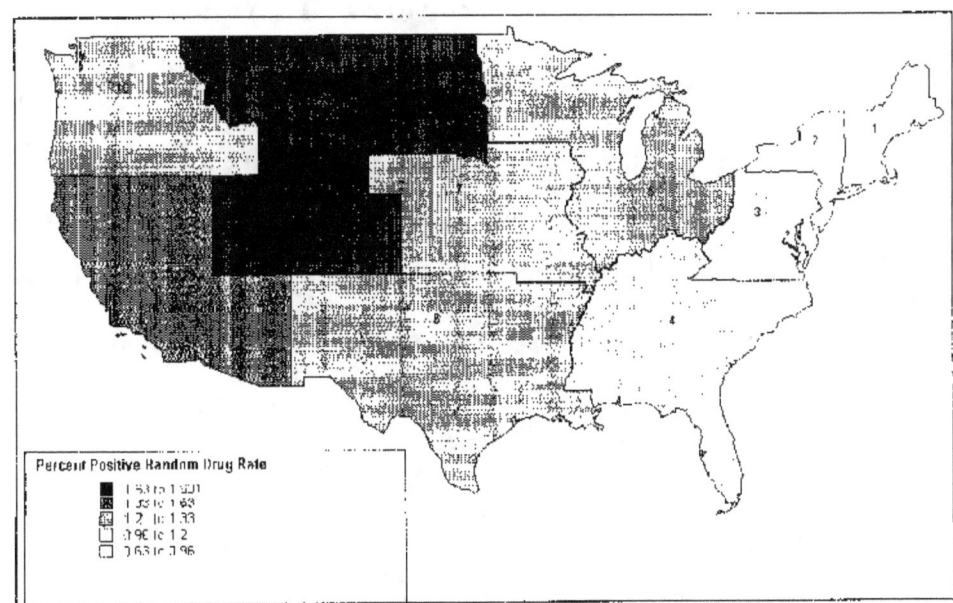

Figure 3-1. Random Drug Test Results by FTA Region

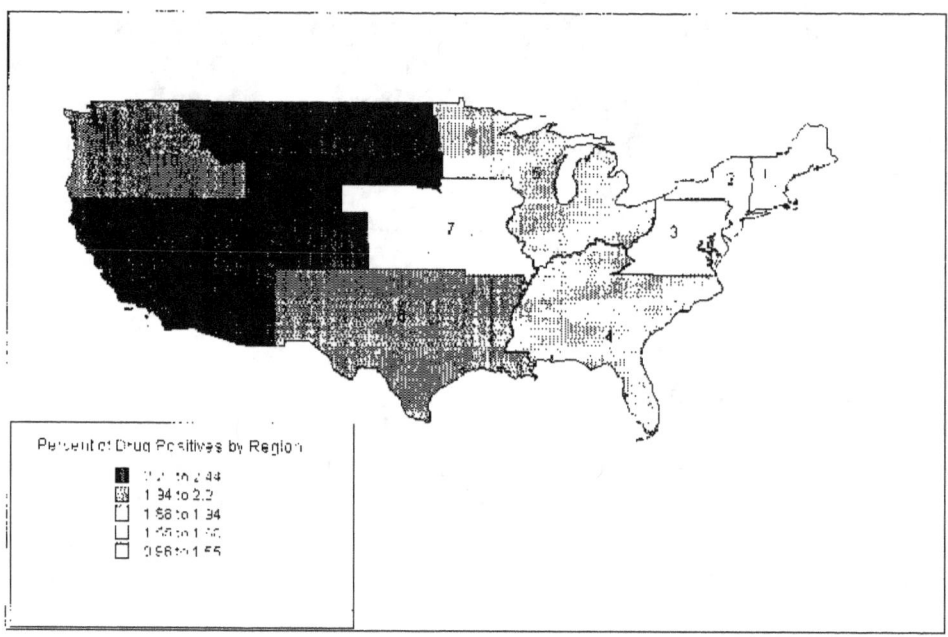

Figure 3-2. Percent of Positives by FTA Region

3.3   Results of Drug Tests Presented by Test Types

Table 3-4 illustrates the drug tests results by comparing transit systems and contractors. The table further categorizes the results by test type and employee category.

Table 3-5 also exhibits the results of the drug tests; however, the data compares employer size, and sorts the results by test type and employee category.

Table 3-4. Drug Test Results by Test Type and Employee Category

Test Type	Transit Systems			Contractors			Totals		
	Number of Specimens Collected	Number of Positive Results	Percent Positive	Number of Specimens Collected	Number of Positive Results	Percent Positive	Number of Specimens Collected	Number of Positive Results	Percent Positive
TOTALS BY TEST TYPE, ALL EMPLOYEE CATEGORIES									
Pre-Employment	44,437	777	1.75%	34,062	1,167	3.43%	78,499	1,944	2.48%
Random	97,185	749	0.77%	24,483	402	1.64%	121,668	1,151	0.95%
Post-Accident	11,772	126	1.07%	3,240	114	3.52%	15,012	240	1.60%
Reasonable Suspicion	822	29	3.53%	252	30	11.90%	1,074	59	5.50%
Return-to-Duty	910	28	3.08%	142	7	4.93%	1,052	35	3.33%
Follow-Up	8,666	127	1.47%	708	27	3.81%	9,374	154	1.64%
TOTALS	163,792	1,836	1.12%	62,887	1,747	2.78%	226,679	3,583	1.59%

Employee Category	Transit Systems			Contractors			Totals		
	Number of Specimens Collected	Number of Positive Results	Percent Positive	Number of Specimens Collected	Number of Positive Results	Percent Positive	Number of Specimens Collected	Number of Positive Results	Percent Positive
PRE-EMPLOYMENT									
Revenue Vehicle Operation	35,781	647	1.81%	30,737	1,081	3.52%	66,518	1,728	2.60%
Revenue Veh. and Equip. Maint.	6,210	102	1.64%	1,784	58	3.25%	7,994	160	2.00%
Revenue Veh. Control/Disp.	1,579	14	0.89%	946	24	2.54%	2,525	38	1.50%
CDL/Non-Revenue Vehicle	382	9	2.36%	70	0	0.0%	452	9	1.99%
Armed Security Personnel	485	5	1.03%	525	4	0.76%	1,010	9	0.89%
RANDOM									
Revenue Vehicle Operation	65,210	498	0.76%	18,877	323	1.71%	84,087	821	.98%
Revenue Veh. and Equip. Maint.	21,010	200	0.95%	3,177	46	1.45%	24,187	246	1.02%
Revenue Veh. Control/Disp.	7,205	26	0.36%	1,793	28	1.56%	8,998	54	0.60%
CDL/Non-Revenue Vehicle	2,332	24	1.03%	266	4	1.50%	2,598	28	1.08%
Armed Security Personnel	1,428	1	0.07%	370	1	0.27%	1,798	2	0.11%

Table 3-4. Drug Test Results by Test Type and Employee Category (continued)

Test Type	Transit Systems			Contractors			Totals		
	Number of Specimens Collected	Number of Positive Results	Percent Positive	Number of Specimens Collected	Number of Positive Results	Percent Positive	Number of Specimens Collected	Number of Positive Results	Percent Positive
POST-ACCIDENT									
Revenue Vehicle Operation	10,791	114	1.06%	3,101	112	3.61%	13,892	226	1.63%
Revenue Veh. and Equip. Maint.	672	11	1.64%	111	2	1.80%	783	13	1.66%
Revenue Veh. Control/Disp.	149	0	0.00%	20	0	0.00%	169	0	0.00%
CDL/Non-Revenue Vehicle	93	1	1.08%	7	0	0.00%	100	1	1.00%
Armed Security Personnel	67	0	0.00%	1	0	0.00%	68	0	0.00%
REASONABLE SUSPICION									
Revenue Vehicle Operation	667	23	3.45%	225	23	10.22%	892	46	5.16%
Revenue Veh. and Equip. Maint.	115	5	4.35%	20	6	30.00%	135	11	8.15%
Revenue Veh. Control/Disp.	24	0	0.00%	5	1	16.67%	30	1	3.33%
CDL/Non-Revenue Vehicle	14	1	7.14%	0	0	0.00%	14	1	7.14%
Armed Security Personnel	2	0	0.00%	1	0	0.00%	3	0	0.00%
RETURN-TO-DUTY									
Revenue Vehicle Operation	654	22	3.36%	110	5	4.55%	764	27	3.53%
Revenue Veh. and Equip. Maint.	202	6	2.97%	21	1	4.76%	223	7	3.14%
Revenue Veh. Control/Disp.	36	0	0.00%	10	1	10.00%	46	1	2.17%
CDL/Non-Revenue Vehicle	17	0	0.00%	1	0	0.00%	18	0	0.00%
Armed Security Personnel	1	0	0.00%	0	0	0.00%	1	0	0.00%
FOLLOW-UP									
Revenue Vehicle Operation	5,033	84	1.67%	479	21	4.38%	5,512	105	1.90%
Revenue Veh. and Equip. Maint.	2,730	38	1.39%	140	4	2.86%	2,870	42	1.46%
Revenue Veh. Control/Disp.	320	2	0.63%	83	1	1.20%	403	3	0.74%
CDL/Non-Revenue Vehicle	540	2	0.37%	6	1	16.67%	546	3	0.55%
Armed Security Personnel	43	1	2.33%	0	0	0.00%	43	1	2.33%

Table 3-5. Drug Test Results by Test Type and Employee Category by Size

Test Type	Large			Small			Rural		
	Number of Specimens Collected	Number of Positive Results	Percent Positive	Number of Specimens Collected	Number of Positive Results	Percent Positive	Number of Specimens Collected	Number of Positive Results	Percent Positive
TOTALS BY TEST TYPE, ALL EMPLOYEE CATEGORIES									
Pre-Employment	58,905	1,606	2.73%	6,436	143	2.22%	3,158	195	1.48%
Random	96,847	920	0.95%	8,963	115	1.28%	15,858	116	0.73%
Post-Accident	12,838	209	1.62%	1158	17	1.47%	956	14	1.46%
Reasonable Suspicion	980	48	4.90%	35	6	17.14%	59	5	8.47%
Return-to-Duty	889	24	2.70%	77	7	9.09%	86	4	4.65%
Follow-Up	9,022	133	1.47%	262	15	5.73%	90	6	6.67%
TOTALS	179,541	2,940	1.64%	16,931	303	1.79%	30,207	340	1.13%

Employee Category	Large			Small			Rural		
	Number of Specimens Collected	Number of Positive Results	Percent Positive	Number of Specimens Collected	Number of Positive Results	Percent Positive	Number of Specimens Collected	Number of Positive Results	Percent Positive
PRE-EMPLOYMENT									
Revenue Vehicle Operation	49,181	1,436	2.92%	5,563	116	2.09%	11,774	176	1.49%
Revenue Veh. and Equip. Maint.	6,894	132	1.91%	630	21	3.33%	470	7	1.49%
Revenue Veh. Control/Disp.	1,541	22	1.43%	206	6	2.91%	778	10	1.29%
CDL/Non-Revenue Vehicle	290	7	2.41%	26	0	0.00%	136	2	1.47%
Armed Security Personnel	999	9	0.90%	11	0	0.00%	0	0	0.00%
RANDOM									
Revenue Vehicle Operation	64,637	648	1.00%	6,633	84	1.27%	12,817	89	0.69%
Revenue Veh. and Equip. Maint.	21,933	210	0.96%	1,262	24	1.90%	992	12	1.21%
Revenue Veh. Control/Disp.	6,408	41	0.64%	844	6	0.71%	1,746	7	0.40%
CDL/Non-Revenue Vehicle	2,101	19	0.90%	194	1	0.52%	303	8	2.64%
Armed Security Personnel	1,768	2	0.11%	30	0	0.00%	0	0	0.00%

Table 3-5. Drug Test Results by Test Type and Employee Category by Size (continued)

Test Type	Large			Small			Rural		
	Number of Specimens Collected	Number of Positive Results	Percent Positive	Number of Specimens Collected	Number of Positive Results	Percent Positive	Number of Specimens Collected	Number of Positive Results	Percent Positive
POST-ACCIDENT									
Revenue Vehicle Operation	11,930	198	1.66%	1,060	14	1.32%	902	14	1.55%
Revenue Veh. and Equip. Maint.	668	10	1.50%	85	3	3.53%	30	0	0.00%
Revenue Veh. Control/Disp.	144	0	0.00%	11	0	0.00%	14	0	0.00%
CDL/Non-Revenue Vehicle	88	1	1.14%	2	0	0.00%	10	0	0.00%
Armed Security Personnel	68	0	0.00%	0	0	0.00%	0	0	0.00%
REASONABLE SUSPICION									
Revenue Vehicle Operation	815	39	4.79%	27	3	11.11%	50	4	8.00%
Revenue Veh. and Equip. Maint.	121	8	6.61%	7	3	42.86%	7	0	0.00%
Revenue Veh. Control/Disp.	30	1	3.33%	0	0	0.00%	0	0	0.00%
CDL/Non-Revenue Vehicle	11	0	0.00%	1	0	0.00%	2	1	50.00%
Armed Security Personnel	3	0	0.00%	0	0	0.00%	0	0	0.00%
RETURN-TO-DUTY									
Revenue Vehicle Operation	638	21	3.29%	61	3	4.92%	65	3	4.62%
Revenue Veh. and Equip. Maint.	196	2	1.02%	13	4	30.77%	14	1	7.14%
Revenue Veh. Control/Disp.	37	1	2.70%	3	0	0.00%	6	0	0.00%
CDL/Non-Revenue Vehicle	17	0	0.00%	0	0	0.00%	1	0	0.00%
Armed Security Personnel	1	0	0.00%	0	0	0.00%	0	0	0.00%
FOLLOW-UP									
Revenue Vehicle Operation	5,254	91	1.73%	198	11	5.56%	60	3	5.00%
Revenue Veh. and Equip. Maint.	2,794	36	1.29%	60	4	6.67%	16	2	12.50%
Revenue Veh. Control/Disp.	386	2	0.52%	3	0	0.00%	14	1	7.14%
CDL/Non-Revenue Vehicle	545	3	0.55%	1	0	0.00%	0	0	0.00%
Armed Security Personnel	43	1	2.33%	0	0	0.00%	0	0	0.00%

3.4   Post-Accident Testing

In cases of certain mass transit accidents, the FTA mandates post-accident testing. Testing is required only when there is a loss of life and when non-fatal accidents occur and employees' performance is a contributing factor.

In order for an incident to be labeled as an accident, the FTA requires four conditions to be met. One, an individual suffers a bodily injury and immediately receives medical attention away from the scene of the accident. Two, the mass transit vehicle or other vehicles involved incur disabling damage as the result of the occurrence and are transported away from the scene by a tow truck or other vehicle. Three, the mass transit vehicle involved is a rail car, trolley car, trolley bus, or vessel, and is removed from revenue service due to the incident. Lastly, the accident renders a loss of life.

Table 3-6 reveals the relationship between the drug positive rates and the number of fatal and non fatal accidents that have occurred. The results of transit systems and contractors are compared in this table.

Table 3-7 also notes the number of fatal and non-fatal accidents with positive drug results. In this table, however, the operators' sizes are compared.

Table 3-8, again, illustrates the amount of accidents that render positive test results. The table further breaks out the results by each FTA region.

Table 3-9, similar to Table 3-5, demonstrates the number of accidents with positive drug test results while comparing transit systems with contractors. The table also provides a comparison of results between employee categories.

Table 3-6. Accidents Which Resulted in a Post-Accident Positive

Employer	Number of Non-Fatal Accidents	Number of Fatal Accidents	Number of Fatalities
Transit Systems	125	1	1
Contractors	114	0	0
Totals	239	1	1

Table 3-7. Accidents Which Resulted in a Post-Accident Positive by Operator Size

Operator Size	Number of Non-Fatal Accidents	Number of Fatal Accidents	Number of Fatalities
Large	209	0	0
Small	16	1	1
Rural	14	0	0
Totals	239	1	1

Table 3-8. Accidents Which Resulted in a Post-Accident Positive by Region

Region	Number of Non-Fatal Accidents	Number of Fatal Accidents	Number of Fatalities
1	6	0	0
2	29	1	1
3	22	0	0
4	20	0	0
5	41	0	0
6	22	0	0
7	10	0	0
8	10	0	0
9	60	0	0
10	19	0	0
Totals	239	1	1

Table 3-9. Post-Accident Drug Test Positives by Employee Category

Employer	Revenue Vehicle Operations	Vehicle and Equip. Maint.	Rev. Vehicle Cntl/Dsptch	CDL/Non Revenue	Armed Security Personnel
Transit Systems	114	11	0	1	0
Contractors	112	2	0	0	0
Totals	226	13	0	1	0

3.5   Distribution of Positive Drug Test Results by Type of Drug

Section 3.5 presents the distribution of positive drug test results for employees who tested positive for one or more of the five prohibited drugs. To be recorded as a positive result, an employee may have tested positive for one drug or a combination of drugs (e.g., marijuana and cocaine). In order to appreciate the seriousness of testing positive for one or more prohibited drugs, this section also describes the effects of each drug and how it inhibits the activities of safety-sensitive employees.

Marijuana is derived from the hemp plant and comes in a variety of colors such as green, brown, and a gray mixture of leaves. THC or delta-9-tetrahydrocannabinol is the primary active chemical in the drug. The drug has adopted the acronym THC for testing purposes.

THC is absorbed quickly into fatty tissues and stored for a long time. The potency and strength of the chemical causes people to use the drug for the mildly tranquilizing, mood and perception-altering effects it produces.

Cocaine is an addictive substance that comes from coca leaves, or is made synthetically. This drug acts as a stimulant to the central nervous system. Cocaine appears as a white powder substance that is inhaled, injected, freebased (smoked), or applied directly to the nasal membrane or gums. Cocaine gives the user a feeling of exhilaration. The chemicals contained in cocaine trick the brain into feeling it has experienced pleasure, when in fact it has not.

Opiates are derived from a sap taken from a seedpod of the plant "papaver somniferum," or poppy plant. Another name used for opiates is narcotic analgesics. General effects of narcotic analgesics include: sedation, slowed reflexes, raspy speech, sluggish movements, slowed breathing, cold skin, and possible vomiting. Its synthetic form known as "designer drug" is even more deadly and addictive.

Phencyclidine or *PCP* was originally developed as an anesthetic, but adverse side effects prevented its use except as a tranquilizer for large animals. In humans, the drug causes people to experience a feeling of disassociation, where the mind feels separated from the body. This can be very upsetting to some people. Some people panic when their own bodily perceptions become distorted. PCP acts as both a depressant and a hallucinogen, and sometimes as a stimulant.

Amphetamines are potent stimulants that may be sniffed, swallowed, snorted, or injected. They induce exhilarating feelings of power, strength, energy, self-assertion, focus, and enhanced motivation. The need to sleep or eat is diminished. The drug induces a sense of aroused euphoria, which may last several hours. Unlike cocaine, the body does not readily break down amphetamines. Thus, feelings are intensified and ephemeral. Subsequently, there is an intense feeling of mental depression and fatigue.

Figures 3-3 to 3-10, and Table 3-10 provide details on the distribution of test results by type of drug.

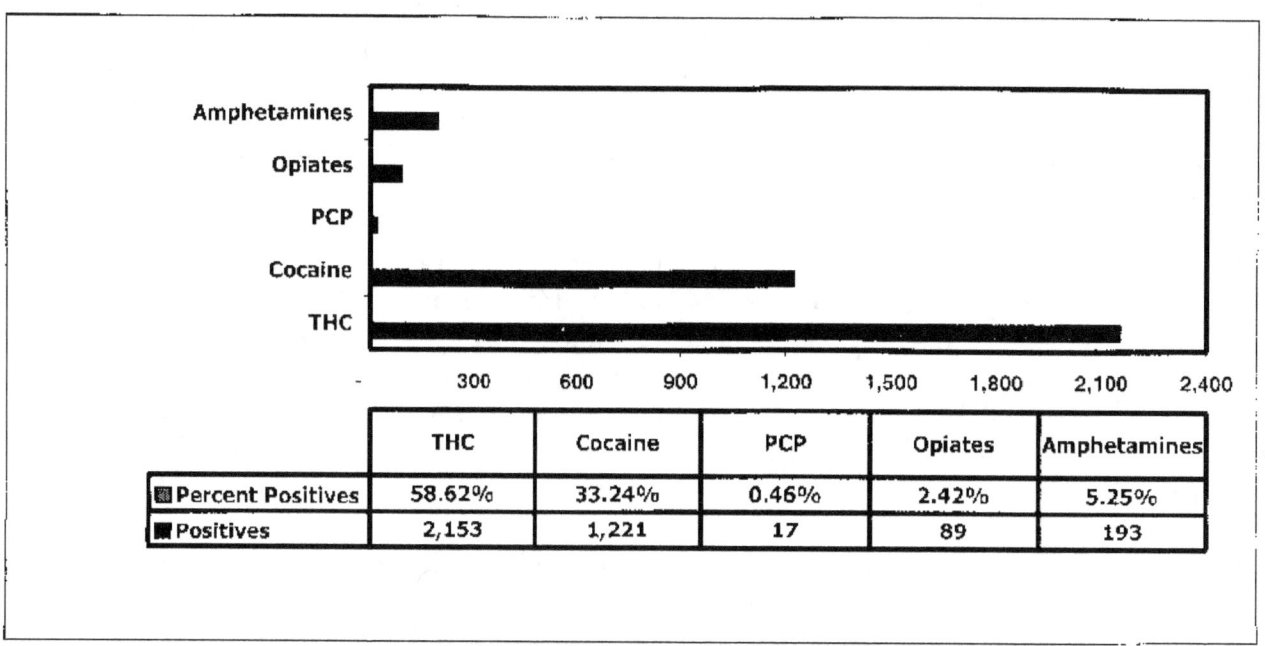

	THC	Cocaine	PCP	Opiates	Amphetamines
Percent Positives	58.62%	33.24%	0.46%	2.42%	5.25%
Positives	2,153	1,221	17	89	193

Figure 3-3. Percentage of Drug Types Detected for All Positive Specimens

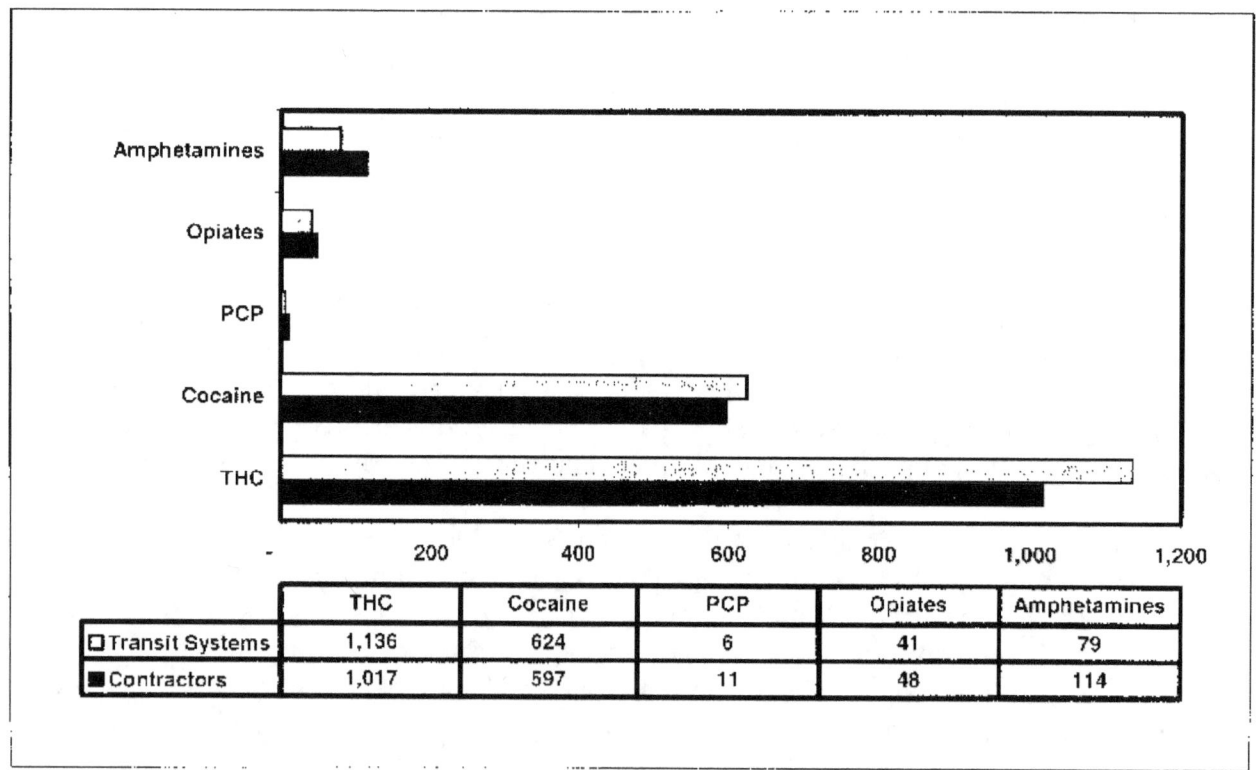

	THC	Cocaine	PCP	Opiates	Amphetamines
Transit Systems	1,136	624	6	41	79
Contractors	1,017	597	11	48	114

Figure 3-4. Number of Positive Specimens by Type of Drug for Each Employer Type

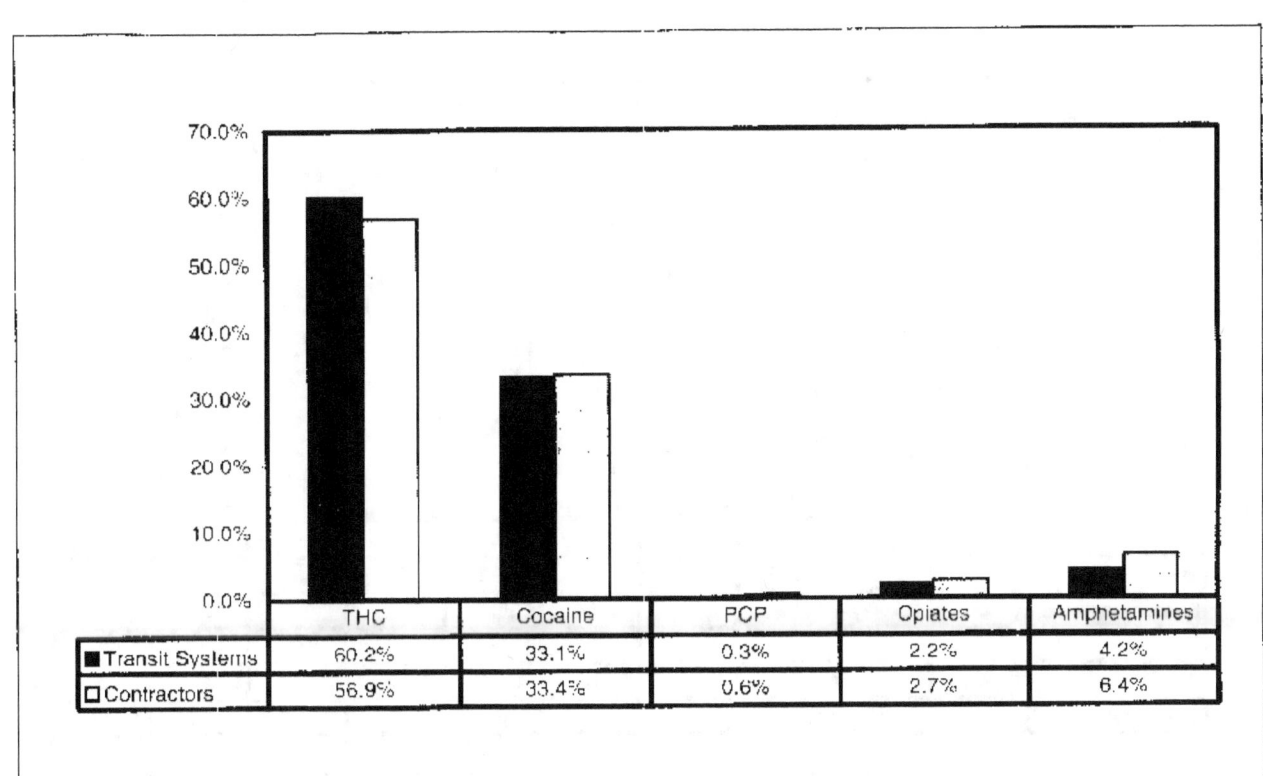

	THC	Cocaine	PCP	Opiates	Amphetamines
■Transit Systems	60.2%	33.1%	0.3%	2.2%	4.2%
□Contractors	56.9%	33.4%	0.6%	2.7%	6.4%

Figure 3-5. Percent of Positive Specimens by Type of Drug for Each Employer Type

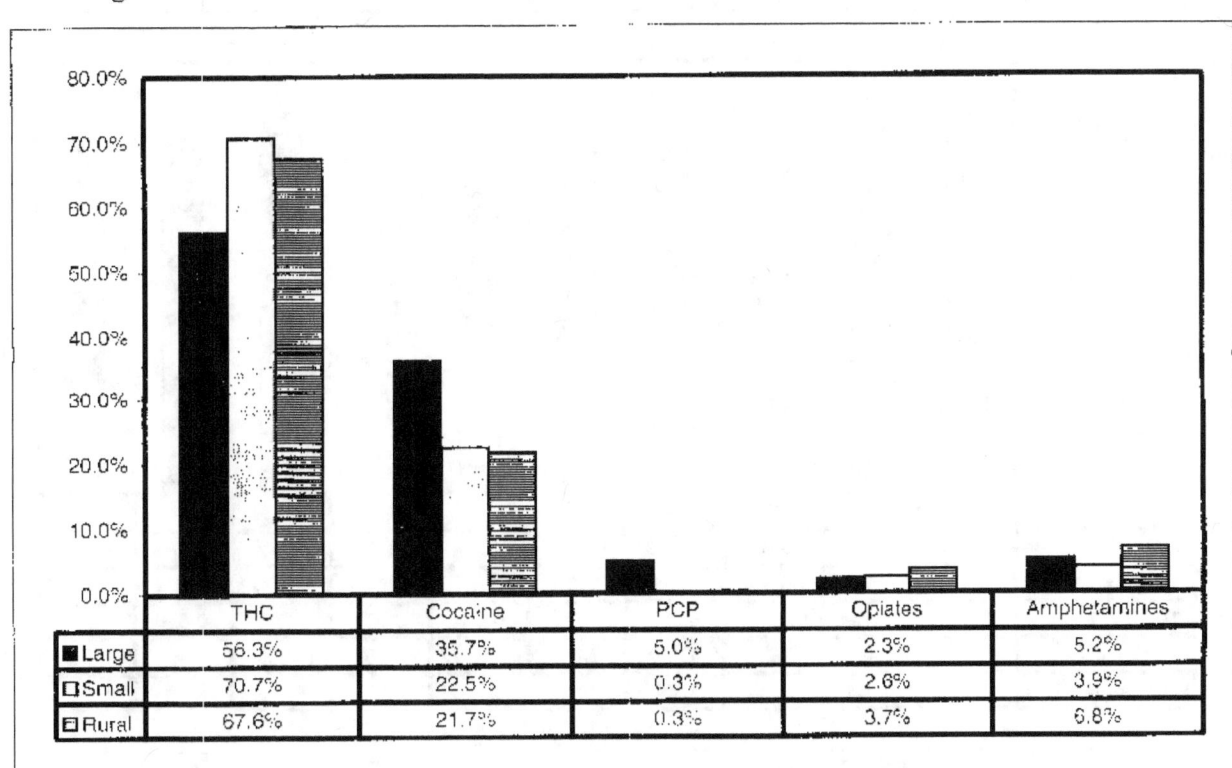

	THC	Cocaine	PCP	Opiates	Amphetamines
■Large	56.3%	35.7%	5.0%	2.3%	5.2%
□Small	70.7%	22.5%	0.3%	2.6%	3.9%
▤Rural	67.6%	21.7%	0.3%	3.7%	6.8%

Figure 3-6. Percent of Positive Specimens by Type of Drug and Operator Size

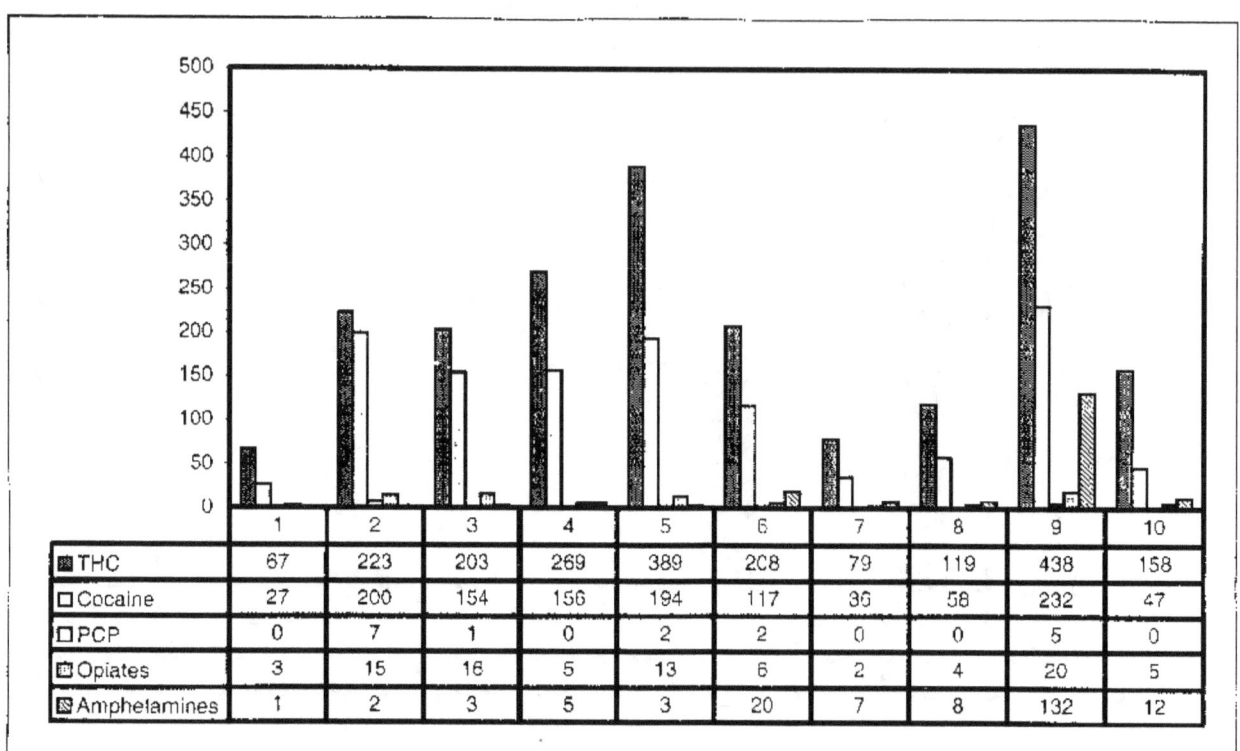

Figure 3-7. Number and Type of Drug by FTA Region

	1	2	3	4	5	6	7	8	9	10
THC	67	223	203	269	389	208	79	119	438	158
Cocaine	27	200	154	156	194	117	36	58	232	47
PCP	0	7	1	0	2	2	0	0	5	0
Opiates	3	15	16	5	13	6	2	4	20	5
Amphetamines	1	2	3	5	3	20	7	8	132	12

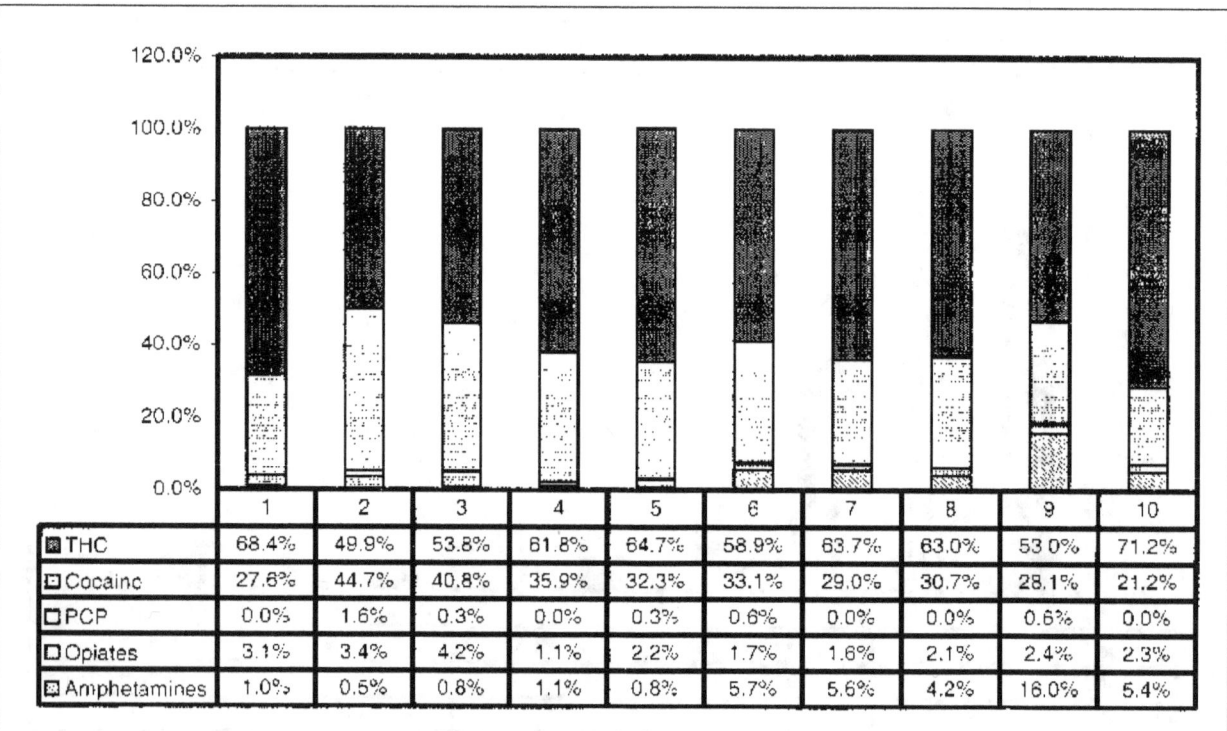

	1	2	3	4	5	6	7	8	9	10
THC	68.4%	49.9%	53.8%	61.8%	64.7%	58.9%	63.7%	63.0%	53.0%	71.2%
Cocaine	27.6%	44.7%	40.8%	35.9%	32.3%	33.1%	29.0%	30.7%	28.1%	21.2%
PCP	0.0%	1.6%	0.3%	0.0%	0.3%	0.6%	0.0%	0.0%	0.6%	0.0%
Opiates	3.1%	3.4%	4.2%	1.1%	2.2%	1.7%	1.6%	2.1%	2.4%	2.3%
Amphetamines	1.0%	0.5%	0.8%	1.1%	0.8%	5.7%	5.6%	4.2%	16.0%	5.4%

Figure 3-8. Percent of Positive Specimens by FTA Region and Type of Drug

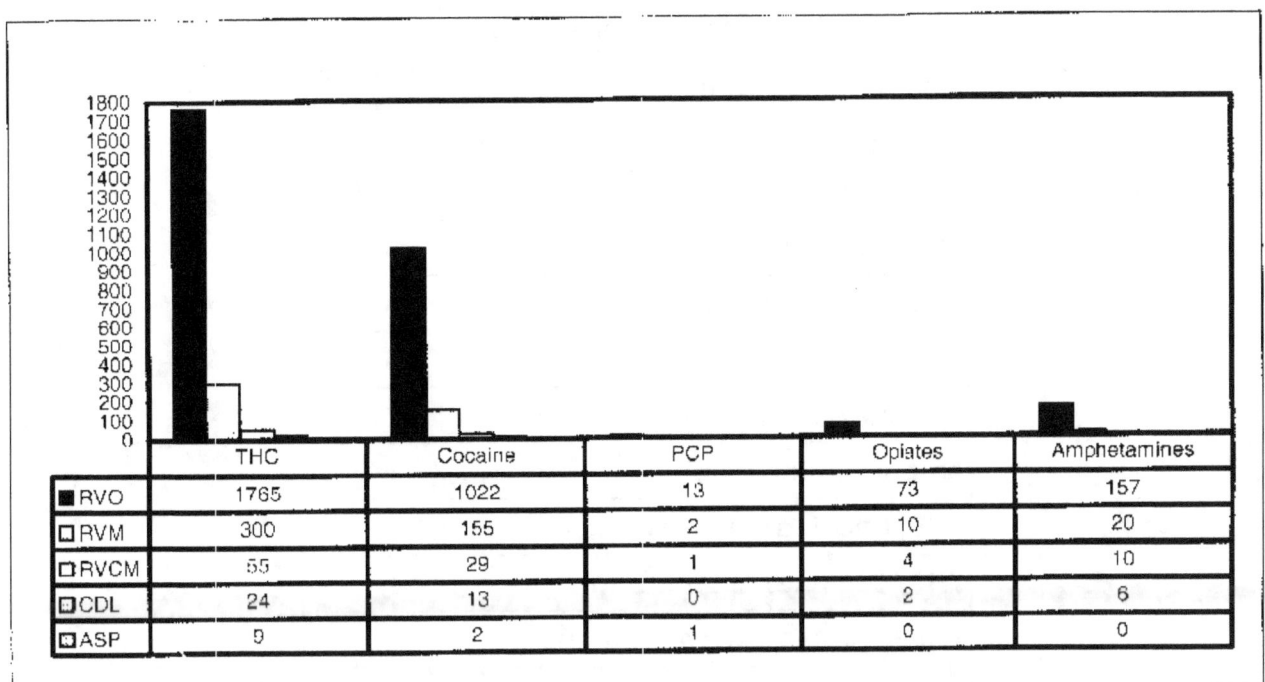

	THC	Cocaine	PCP	Opiates	Amphetamines
■ RVO	1765	1022	13	73	157
□ RVM	300	155	2	10	20
□ RVCM	55	29	1	4	10
□ CDL	24	13	0	2	6
□ ASP	9	2	1	0	0

Figure 3-9. Number of Positive Specimens by Employee Category and Type of Drug

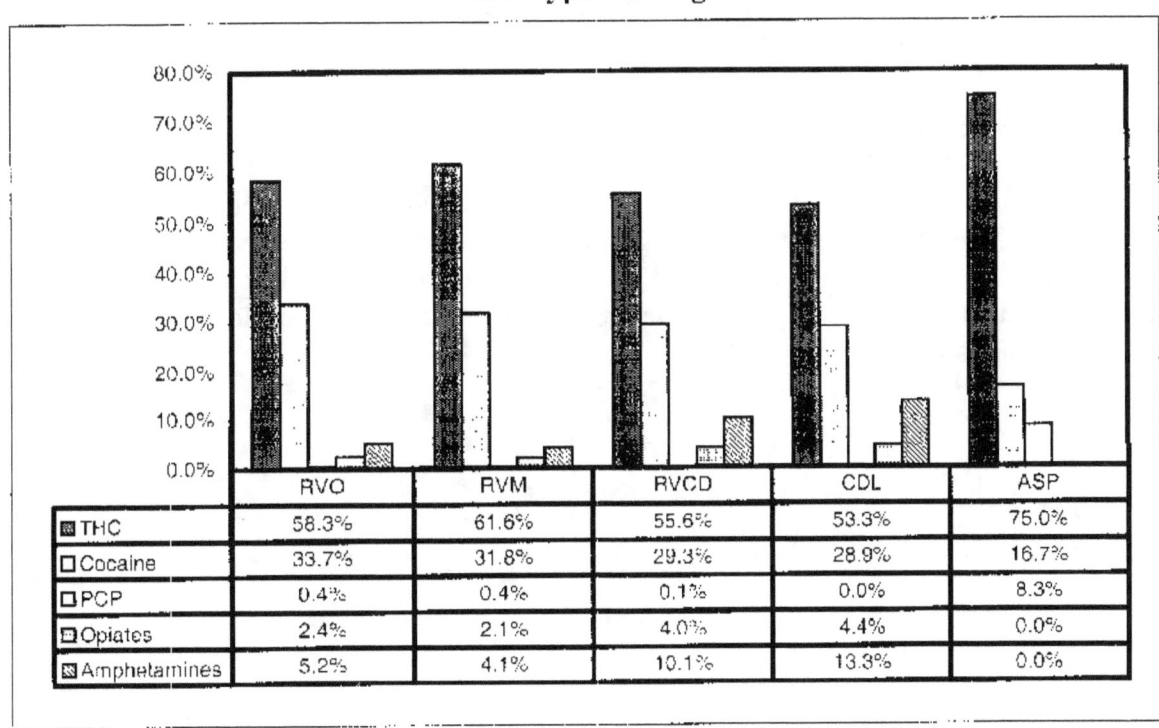

	RVO	RVM	RVCD	CDL	ASP
■ THC	58.3%	61.6%	55.6%	53.3%	75.0%
□ Cocaine	33.7%	31.8%	29.3%	28.9%	16.7%
□ PCP	0.4%	0.4%	0.1%	0.0%	8.3%
□ Opiates	2.4%	2.1%	4.0%	4.4%	0.0%
▨ Amphetamines	5.2%	4.1%	10.1%	13.3%	0.0%

Figure 3-10. Percent of Positive Specimens by Type of Drug and Employee Category

Table 3-10. Multiple Drug Combinations

Drug Combination	Number of Specimens
THC/Cocaine	20
THC/PCP	1
THC/Opiates	3
THC/Amphetamines	5
Cocaine/Opiates	3
Cocaine/Amphetamines	2
Amphetamines/PCP	1
THC/Cocaine/Opiates	5
THC/Cocaine/Amphetamines	1
THC/Opiates/Amphetamines	1
Opiates/Amphetamines	2
PCP/Amphetamines	1
Totals	45

3.6 Drug Test Refusals

Drug test refusals are based upon the number of employees, who when directed to provide specimens for testing, refuse to be tested. In 2000, there were 126 reported cases of covered employees refusing random drug testing and 69 cases of a covered employee refusing a non-random drug test. These refusals reflect .09 percent of the total number of drug tests attempted. For more information, see Figure 3-11.

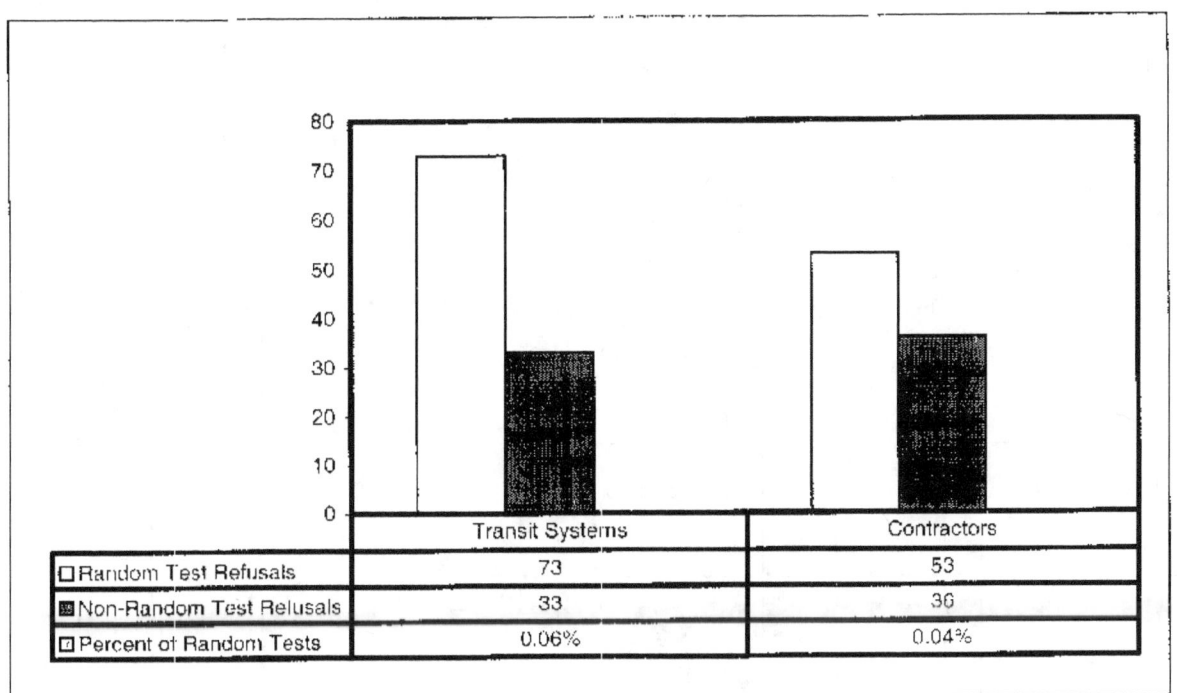

	Transit Systems	Contractors
☐ Random Test Refusals	73	53
■ Non-Random Test Refusals	33	36
☐ Percent of Random Tests	0.06%	0.04%

Figure 3-11. Drug Test Refusals

3.7   Return-to-Duty Positive Rate

Table 3-11 represents the total number of employees who returned to duty after receiving a positive drug test or after refusing to take a drug test. The consequences of refusing a drug test and for testing positive are synonymous.

Table 3-11. Number of Covered Employees Who Returned-to-Duty

Employer Type	Returned-to-Duty	Percent of Total
Transit Systems	415	84.0
Contractors	79	16.0
Totals	**494**	**100.0**

3.8   Results of Drug Tests Presented by Employee Category

Tables 3-12 and 3-13 illustrate the drug test results by employee category. Specifically, Table 3-12 compares the results of transit systems and contractors. Table 3-13 presents drug test results by employee category for large, small, and rural systems.

2000 Annual Report

Table 3-12. Drug Test Results by Employee Category and Test Type by Transit System and Contractor

Employee Category	Transit Systems			Contractors			Totals		
	Number of Specimens Collected	Number of Positive Results	Percent Positive	Number of Specimens Collected	Number of Positive Results	Percent Positive	Number of Specimens Collected	Number of Positive Results	Percent Positive
TOTALS BY EMPLOYEE CATEGORY, ALL TEST TYPES									
Revenue Vehicle Operation	118,136	1,388	1.17%	53,529	1,565	2.92%	171,665	2,953	1.72%
Revenue Veh. and Equip. Maint.	30,939	362	1.17%	5,253	117	2.23%	36,192	479	1.32%
Revenue Veh. Control/Disp.	9,313	42	0.45%	2,858	55	1.92%	12,171	97	0.80%
CDL/Non-Revenue Vehicle	3,378	37	1.10%	350	5	1.43%	3,728	42	1.13%
Armed Security Personnel	2,026	7	0.35%	897	5	0.56%	2,923	12	0.41%
TOTALS	**163,792**	**1,836**	**1.12%**	**62,887**	**1,747**	**2.78%**	**226,679**	**3,583**	**1.58%**

Test Type	Transit Systems			Contractors			Totals		
	Number of Specimens Collected	Number of Positive Results	Percent Positive	Number of Specimens Collected	Number of Positive Results	Percent Positive	Number of Specimens Collected	Number of Positive Results	Percent Positive
REVENUE VEHICLE OPERATOR									
Pre-Employment	35,781	647	1.81%	30,737	1,081	3.52%	66,518	1,728	2.51%
Random	65,210	498	0.76%	18,877	323	1.71%	84,087	821	1.01%
Post-Accident	10,791	114	1.06%	3,101	112	3.61%	13,892	226	1.52%
Reasonable Suspicion	667	23	3.45%	225	23	10.22%	892	46	9.79%
Return-to-Duty	654	22	3.36%	110	5	4.55%	764	27	3.93%
Follow-Up	5,033	84	1.67%	479	21	4.38%	5,512	105	1.80%
REVENUE VEHICLE AND EQUIPMENT MAINTENANCE									
Pre-Employment	6,210	102	1.64%	1,784	58	3.25%	7,994	160	2.00%
Random	21,010	200	0.95%	3,177	46	1.45%	24,187	246	1.02%
Post-Accident	672	11	1.64%	111	2	1.80%	783	13	1.66%
Reasonable Suspicion	115	5	4.35%	20	6	30.00%	135	11	8.15%
Return-to-Duty	202	6	2.97%	21	1	4.76%	223	7	3.14%
Follow-Up	2,730	38	1.39%	140	4	2.86%	2,870	42	1.46%

Table 3-12. Drug Test Results by Employee Category and Test Type by Transit System and Contractor (continued)

Test Type	Transit Systems			Contractors			Totals		
	Number of Specimens Collected	Number of Positive Results	Percent Positive	Number of Specimens Collected	Number of Positive Results	Percent Positive	Number of Specimens Collected	Number of Positive Results	Percent Positive
REVENUE VEHICLE CONTROL/ DISPATCH									
Pre-Employment	1,579	14	0.89%	946	24	2.54%	2,525	38	1.50%
Random	7,205	26	0.36%	1,793	28	1.56%	8,998	54	0.60%
Post-Accident	149	0	0.00%	20	0	0.00%	169	0	0.00%
Reasonable Suspicion	24	0	0.00%	6	1	16.67%	30	1	3.33%
Return-to-Duty	36	0	0.00%	10	1	10.00%	46	1	2.17%
Follow-Up	320	2	0.63%	83	1	1.20%	403	3	0.74%
CDL/NON-REVENUE VEHICLE									
Pre-Employment	382	9	2.36%	70	0	0.00%	452	9	1.99%
Random	2,332	24	1.03%	266	4	1.50%	2,598	28	1.08%
Post-Accident	93	1	1.08%	7	0	0.00%	100	1	1.00%
Reasonable Suspicion	14	1	7.14%	0	0	0.00%	14	1	7.14%
Return-to-Duty	17	0	0.00%	1	0	0.00%	18	0	0.00%
Follow-Up	540	2	0.37%	6	1	16.67%	546	3	0.55%
ARMED SECURITY PERSONNEL									
Pre-Employment	485	5	1.03%	525	4	0.76%	1,010	9	0.89%
Random	1,428	1	0.07%	370	1	0.27%	1,798	2	0.11%
Post-Accident	67	0	0.00%	1	0	0.00%	68	0	0.00%
Reasonable Suspicion	2	0	0.00%	1	0	0.00%	3	0	0.00%
Return-to-Duty	1	0	0.00%	0	0	0.00%	1	0	0.00%
Follow-Up	43	1	2.33%	0	0	0.00%	43	1	2.33%

Table 3-13. Drug Test Results by Employee Category and Test Type by Size

TOTALS BY EMPLOYEE CATEGORY, ALL TEST TYPES

Employee Category	Large			Small			Rural		
	Number of Specimens Collected	Number of Positive Results	Percent Positive	Number of Specimens Collected	Number of Positive Results	Percent Positive	Number of Specimens Collected	Number of Positive Results	Percent Positive
Revenue Vehicle Operation	132,455	2,433	1.84%	13,542	231	1.71%	25,668	289	1.13%
Revenue Veh. and Equip. Maint.	34,606	398	1.22%	2,057	59	2.87%	1,529	22	1.44%
Revenue Veh. Control/Disp.	8,546	67	0.78%	1,067	12	1.12%	2,558	18	0.70%
CDL/Non-Revenue Vehicle	3,052	30	0.98%	224	1	0.45%	452	11	2.43%
Armed Security Personnel	2,882	12	0.42%	41	0	0.00%	0	0	0.00%
TOTALS	179,541	2,940	1.64%	16,931	303	1.79%	30,207	340	1.13%

Test Type	Large			Small			Rural		
	Number of Specimens Collected	Number of Positive Results	Percent Positive	Number of Specimens Collected	Number of Positive Results	Percent Positive	Number of Specimens Collected	Number of Positive Results	Percent Positive
REVENUE VEHICLE OPERATOR									
Pre-Employment	49,181	1,436	2.92%	5,563	116	2.09%	11,774	176	1.49%
Random	64,637	648	1.00%	6,633	84	1.27%	12,817	89	0.69%
Post-Accident	11,930	198	1.66%	1,060	14	1.32%	902	14	1.55%
Reasonable Suspicion	815	39	4.79%	27	3	11.11%	50	4	8.00%
Return-to-Duty	638	21	3.29%	61	3	4.92%	65	3	4.62%
Follow-Up	5,254	91	1.73%	198	11	5.56%	60	3	5.00%
REVENUE VEHICLE AND EQUIPMENT MAINTENANCE									
Pre-Employment	6,894	132	1.91%	630	21	3.33%	470	7	1.49%
Random	21,933	210	0.96%	1,262	24	1.90%	992	12	1.21%
Post-Accident	668	10	1.50%	85	3	3.53%	30	0	0.00%
Reasonable Suspicion	121	8	6.61%	7	3	42.86%	7	0	0.00%
Return-to-Duty	196	2	1.02%	13	4	30.77%	14	1	7.14%
Follow-Up	2,794	36	1.29%	60	4	6.67%	16	2	12.5%

Table 3-13. Drug Test Results by Employee Category and Test Type by Size (continued)

Test Type	Large			Small			Rural		
	Number of Specimens Collected	Number of Positive Results	Percent Positive	Number of Specimens Collected	Number of Positive Results	Percent Positive	Number of Specimens Collected	Number of Positive Results	Percent Positive
REVENUE VEHICLE CONTROL/ DISPATCH									
Pre-Employment	1,541	22	1.43%	206	6	2.91%	778	10	1.29%
Random	6,408	41	0.64%	844	6	0.71%	1,746	7	0.40%
Post-Accident	144	0	0.00%	11	0	0.00%	14	0	0.00%
Reasonable Suspicion	30	1	3.33%	0	0	0.00%	0	0	0.00%
Return-to-Duty	37	1	2.70%	3	0	0.00%	6	0	0.00%
Follow-Up	386	2	0.52%	3	0	0.00%	14	1	7.14%
CDL/NON-REVENUE VEHICLE									
Pre-Employment	290	7	2.41%	26	0	0.00%	136	2	1.47%
Random	2,101	19	0.90%	194	1	0.52%	303	8	2.64%
Post-Accident	88	1	1.14%	2	0	0.00%	10	0	0.00%
Reasonable Suspicion	11	0	0.00%	1	0	0.00%	2	1	50.00%
Return-to-Duty	17	0	0.00%	0	0	0.00%	1	0	0.00%
Follow-Up	545	3	0.55%	1	0	0.00%	0	0	0.00%
ARMED SECURITY PERSONNEL									
Pre-Employment	999	9	0.90%	11	0	0.00%	0	0	0.00%
Random	1,768	2	0.11%	30	0	0.00%	3	0	0.00%
Post-Accident	68	0	0.00%	0	0	0.00%	0	0	0.00%
Reasonable Suspicion	3	0	0.00%	0	0	0.00%	0	0	0.00%
Return-to-Duty	1	0	0.00%	0	0	0.00%	0	0	0.00%
Follow-Up	43	1	2.33%	0	0	0.00%	0	0	0.00%

4. ALCOHOL TEST RESULTS

Chapter 4 provides background information on the alcohol testing procedures and a summary of the 2000 alcohol test results. The chapter also discusses results of random alcohol testing for transit systems and contracts, by employer size, and by region.

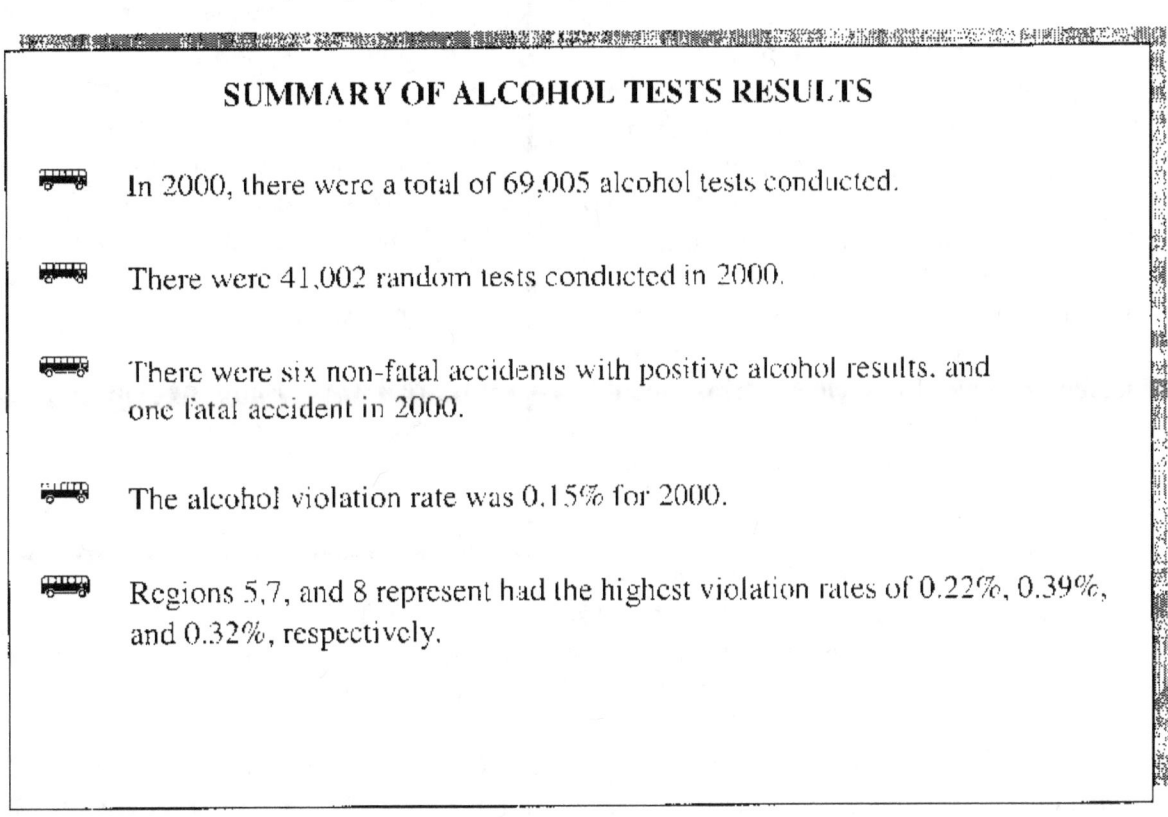

SUMMARY OF ALCOHOL TESTS RESULTS

- In 2000, there were a total of 69,005 alcohol tests conducted.

- There were 41,002 random tests conducted in 2000.

- There were six non-fatal accidents with positive alcohol results, and one fatal accident in 2000.

- The alcohol violation rate was 0.15% for 2000.

- Regions 5,7, and 8 represent had the highest violation rates of 0.22%, 0.39%, and 0.32%, respectively.

Employees of FTA-funded agencies are prohibited from using alcohol while performing safety-sensitive functions. Specifically, employees who hold safety-sensitive functions must not consume alcohol 4 hours prior to reporting to work. In cases when employees violate this regulation and the employer is aware of it, the agency must give the employee the opportunity to acknowledge use of alcohol at the time he or she arrives to duty. An alcohol test must be administered if the employee claims to be able to perform his or her safety-sensitive functions. In the case of a FTA-defined accident, an employee cannot drink alcohol for 8 hours following the incident unless they have been tested prior to this 8-hour time period.

An employee with an alcohol concentration of ≥ 0.02 but < 0.04 must be removed from his or her safety-sensitive position for 8 hours or until a re-test shows an alcohol concentration of < 0.02.

An employee with an alcohol concentration of ≥ 0.04 must be removed from his or her safety-sensitive position, be told about educational and treatment programs available, and be referred to a substance abuse professional.

Figure 4-1. Consequences of an Alcohol Test for FTA-Covered Employees

A post-accident test is required for prohibited drugs and alcohol, following certain mass transit accidents. These accidents include those in which a death occurs, medical treatment away from the scene of the incident is required, or one or more of the vehicles involved incurs disabling damage.

The FTA provides different sets of consequences (see Figure 4-1) should an alcohol confirmation test show that an employee's alcohol concentration is (1) ≥ 0.02 but < 0.04, or (2) ≥ 0.04.

The alcohol concentration level is the amount of alcohol in a volume of breath expressed in terms of grams of alcohol per 210 liters of breath. Alcohol tests are conducted in two parts: a screening test, followed by a confirmation test for those employees for whom the screening test result indicates an alcohol concentration ≥ 0.02.

The data collected by the FTA from transit systems and contractors includes information on the number of screening tests conducted, the number of confirmation tests conducted, and the results from these confirmation tests. In this report, the alcohol test results are derived from the number of screening tests conducted that are found to be ≥ 0.04. The number of screening tests is used to better reflect accurate testing percentages. Because confirmation tests are only performed once a screening test has resulted in ≥ 0.02, to report results ≥ 0.04 of confirmation tests would result in high and misleading percentages.

Table 4-1 shows the percent of alcohol forms submitted by transit systems and contractors with at least one positive test result in 2000.

Table 4-1. Percent of Alcohol Forms Received for 2000 with at Least One Positive Test Result

Employer Type	Number of Employers	Number 0.02 - 0.04	Percent with a Test 0.02 – 0.04	Number ≥ 0.04	Percent with a Positive
Transit Systems	1,700	38	2.24%	58	3.41%
Contractors	957	12	1.25%	31	3.24%
Totals	**2,657**	**50**	**1.88%**	**89**	**3.35%**

Table 4-2 shows the results of random alcohol testing for transit systems and contractors. Random alcohol testing was the type of test conducted most frequently; 41,002 tests out of 69,005 total tests. Although Table 4-2 shows the number of random "positives" for alcohol tests ≥ 0.02 but < 0.04, for reporting purposes verified positives are considered > 0.04. Table 4-3 provides random alcohol test results at both levels by size. The positive random alcohol test rate in 2000 was 0.10%.

Table 4-2. Random Alcohol Test Results at Both Levels for Transit Systems and Contractors

Employer Type	Total Screens	Number 0.02 - 0.04	Number ≥ 0.04	Percent 0.02 - 0.04	Percent ≥ 0.04
Transit Systems	33,300	30	33	0.09%	0.10%
Contractors	7,702	6	9	0.08%	0.12%
Totals	**41,002**	**36**	**42**	**0.09%**	**0.10%**

Table 4-3. Random Alcohol Test Results at Both Levels by Size

Size	Total Screens	Number 0.02 - 0.04	Number ≥ 0.04	Percent 0.02 - 0.04	Percent ≥ 0.04
Large	33,241	35	34	0.11%	0.10%
Small	2,709	1	1	0.04%	0.04%
Rural	5,052	0	7	0.00%	0.14%
Totals	**41,002**	**36**	**42**	**0.09%**	**0.10%**

4.1   Alcohol Tests by FTA Region

This section reports alcohol test results by FTA region. A list of the states in each FTA region can be found in Appendix A. As shown in Figure 4 2, of the 10 FTA regions, Regions 7 and 8 had the highest percent of specimens that tested positive for alcohol. Regions 5 and 8 had the highest percent of positive random alcohol rates, as shown in Figure 4-3. Table 4-4 provides the actual numbers for random alcohol test results at both levels by region.

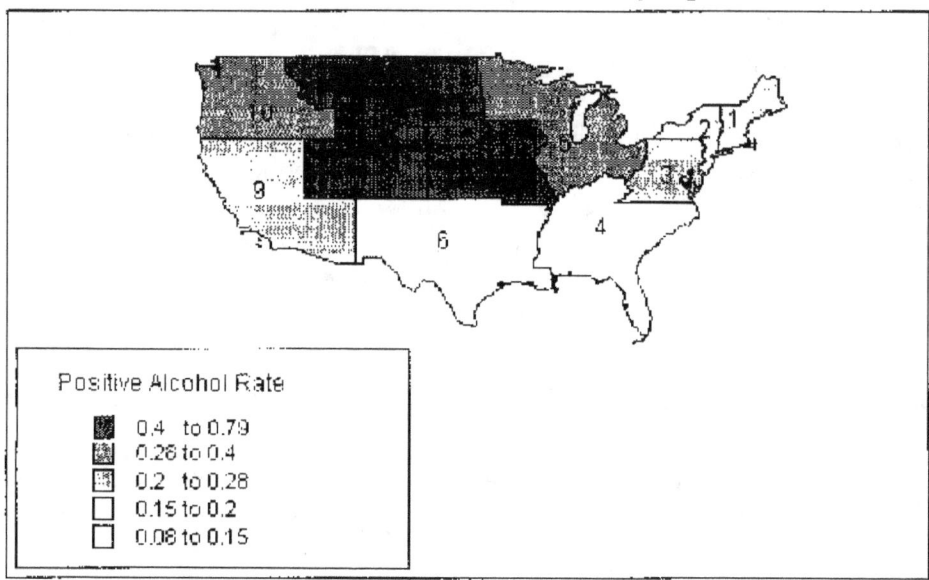

Figure 4-2. Positive Alcohol Rates by Region

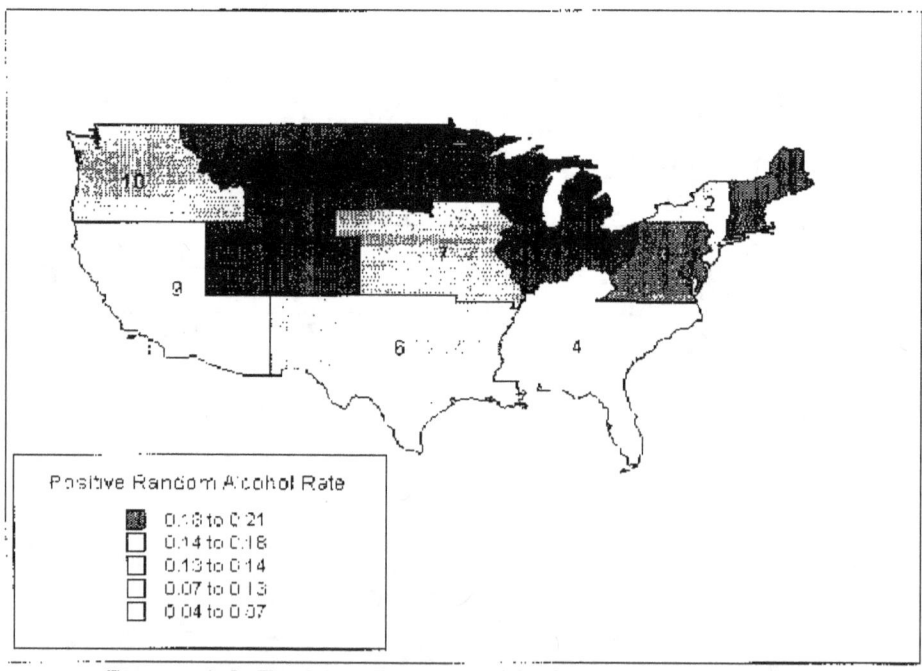

Figure 4-3. Positive Random Alcohol Rates by Region

Table 4-4. Random Alcohol Test Results at Both Levels by Region

Region	Total Screens	Number 0.02 - 0.04	Number ≥ 0.04	Percent 0.02 - 0.04	Percent ≥ 0.04
1	1,787	1	3	0.06%	0.17%
2	8,448	7	8	0.08%	0.09%
3	6,486	6	9	0.09%	0.14%
4	6,470	0	3	0.00%	0.05%
5	5,079	9	9	0.18%	0.18%
6	4,550	3	3	0.07%	0.07%
7	761	0	1	0.00%	0.13%
8	937	0	2	0.00%	0.21%
9	4,905	9	2	0.18%	0.04%
10	1,579	1	2	0.06%	0.13%
Totals	**41,002**	**36**	**42**	**0.09%**	**0.10%**

4.2   Results of Alcohol Testing by Test Type and Employee Category

Alcohol test information was required from transit systems and their contractors for five test types: random, post-accident, reasonable suspicion, return-to-duty, and follow-up. Although the requirement to conduct pre-employment testing was suspended by the FTA as of May 10, 1995, some employers still provide the test and the results.

Table 4-5 presents the alcohol test results by test type and by employee category for transit systems and contractors, and identifies the combined totals. Table 4-6 presents the alcohol test results by test type and employee category for large, small, and rural systems. Table 4-7 presents alcohol testing information by employee category and test type for transit systems, contractors, and totals. Table 4-8 presents the alcohol test results by employee category and test type for large, small, and rural systems and their combined totals.

Table 4-5. Alcohol Test Results by Test Type and Employee Category by Transit System and Contractor

	Transit Systems			Contractors			Totals		
Test Type	Number of Screening Tests	Number of Results ≥ 0.04	Percent ≥ 0.04	Number of Screening Tests	Number of Results ≥ 0.04	Percent ≥ 0.04	Number of Screening Tests	Number of Results ≥ 0.04	Percent ≥ 0.04
TOTALS BY TEST TYPE, ALL EMPLOYEE CATEGORIES									
Pre-Employment	3,745	2	0.05%	2,351	0	0.00%	6,096	2	0.03%
Random	33,300	33	0.10%	7,702	9	0.12%	41,002	42	0.10%
Post-Accident	11,179	5	0.04%	2,604	0	0.00%	13,783	5	0.04%
Reasonable Suspicion	809	53	6.55%	233	28	12.02%	1,042	81	7.77%
Return-to-Duty	546	0	0.00%	52	0	0.00%	598	0	0.00%
Follow-Up	5,962	9	0.15%	522	1	0.19%	6,484	10	0.15%
TOTALS	**55,541**	**102**	**0.18%**	**13,464**	**38**	**0.28%**	**69,005**	**140**	**0.20%**

	Transit Systems			Contractors			Totals		
Employee Category	Number of Screening Tests	Number of Results ≥ 0.04	Percent ≥ 0.04	Number of Screening Tests	Number of Results ≥ 0.04	Percent ≥ 0.04	Number of Screening Tests	Number of Results ≥ 0.04	Percent ≥ 0.04
PRE-EMPLOYMENT									
Revenue Vehicle Operations	3,107	2	0.06%	2,030	0	0.00%	5,137	2	0.04%
Vehicle and Equipment Maintenance	389	0	0.00%	166	0	0.00%	555	0	0.00%
Revenue Vehicle Control/Dispatch	159	0	0.00%	87	0	0.00%	246	0	0.00%
CDL/Non-Revenue Vehicle	57	0	0.00%	1	0	0.00%	58	0	0.00%
Armed Security Personnel	33	0	0.00%	67	0	0.00%	100	0	0.00%
RANDOM									
Revenue Vehicle Operations	22,039	19	0.09%	5,715	6	0.10%	27,754	25	0.09%
Vehicle and Equipment Maintenance	7,052	7	0.10%	1,185	3	0.25%	8,237	10	0.12%
Revenue Vehicle Control/Dispatch	2,122	4	0.19%	588	0	0.00%	2,710	4	0.15%
CDL/Non-Revenue Vehicle	1,399	3	0.21%	53	0	0.00%	1,452	3	0.21%
Armed Security Personnel	688	0	0.00%	161	0	0.00%	849	0	0.00%

Table 4-5. Alcohol Test Results by Test Type and Employee Category by Transit System and Contractor (continued)

Employee Category	Transit Systems			Contractors			Totals		
	Number of Screening Tests	Number of Results ≥ 0.04	Percent ≥ 0.04	Number of Screening Tests	Number of Results ≥ 0.04	Percent ≥ 0.04	Number of Screening Tests	Number of Results ≥ 0.04	Percent ≥ 0.04
POST-ACCIDENT									
Revenue Vehicle Operations	10,239	4	0.04%	2,492	0	0.00%	12,731	4	0.03%
Vehicle and Equipment Maintenance	638	0	0.00%	96	0	0.00%	734	0	0.00%
Revenue Vehicle Control/Dispatch	143	0	0.00%	11	0	0.00%	154	0	0.00%
CDL/Non-Revenue Vehicle	92	1	1.09%	4	0	0.00%	96	1	1.04%
Armed Security Personnel	67	0	0.00%	1	0	0.00%	68	0	0.00%
REASONABLE SUSPICION									
Revenue Vehicle Operations	659	40	6.07%	217	24	11.06%	876	64	7.31%
Vehicle and Equipment Maintenance	112	9	8.04%	9	2	22.22%	121	11	9.09%
Revenue Vehicle Control/Dispatch	23	3	13.04%	7	2	28.57%	30	5	16.67%
CDL/Non-Revenue Vehicle	13	1	7.69%	0	0	0.00%	13	1	7.69%
Armed Security Personnel	2	0	0.00%	0	0	0.00%	2	0	0.00%
RETURN-TO-DUTY									
Revenue Vehicle Operations	380	0	0.00%	37	0	0.00%	417	0	0.00%
Vehicle and Equipment Maintenance	138	0	0.00%	13	0	0.00%	151	0	0.00%
Revenue Vehicle Control/Dispatch	16	0	0.00%	2	0	0.00%	18	0	0.00%
CDL/Non-Revenue Vehicle	11	0	0.00%	0	0	0.00%	11	0	0.00%
Armed Security Personnel	1	0	0.00%	0	0	0.00%	1	0	0.00%
FOLLOW-UP									
Revenue Vehicle Operations	3,457	8	0.23%	328	1	0.30%	3,785	9	0.24%
Vehicle and Equipment Maintenance	1,923	1	0.05%	133	0	0.00%	2,056	1	0.05%
Revenue Vehicle Control/Dispatch	251	0	0.00%	61	0	0.00%	312	0	0.00%
CDL/Non-Revenue Vehicle	300	0	0.00%	0	0	0.00%	300	0	0.00%
Armed Security Personnel	31	0	0.00%	0	0	0.00%	31	0	0.00%

Table 4-6. Alcohol Test Results by Test Type and Employee Category by Size

Test Type	Large			Small			Rural		
	Number of Screening Tests	Number of Results ≥ 0.04	Percent ≥ 0.04	Number of Screening Tests	Number of Results ≥ 0.04	Percent ≥ 0.04	Number of Screening Tests	Number of Results ≥ 0.04	Percent ≥ 0.04
TOTALS BY TEST TYPE, ALL EMPLOYEE CATEGORIES									
Pre-Employment	4,016	1	0.02%	944	0	0.00%	1,136	1	0.02%
Random	33,241	34	0.10%	2,709	1	0.04%	5,052	7	0.02%
Post-Accident	12,062	4	0.03%	991	0	0.00%	724	1	0.00%
Reasonable Suspicion	960	65	6.77%	34	7	20.59%	48	9	11.11%
Return-to-Duty	564	0	0.00%	18	0	0.00%	16	0	0.00%
Follow-Up	6,369	10	0.16%	65	0	0.00%	50	0	0.00%
TOTALS	57,212	114	0.20%	4,767	8	0.17%	7,026	18	0.26%

Employee Category	Large			Small			Rural		
	Number of Screening Tests	Number of Results ≥ 0.04	Percent ≥ 0.04	Number of Screening Tests	Number of Results ≥ 0.04	Percent ≥ 0.04	Number of Screening Tests	Number of Results ≥ 0.04	Percent ≥ 0.04
PRE-EMPLOYMENT									
Revenue Vehicle Operations	3,382	1	0.03%	779	0	0.00%	976	1	0.10%
Vehicle and Equipment Maintenance	401	0	0.00%	115	0	0.00%	39	0	0.00%
Revenue Vehicle Control/Dispatch	107	0	0.00%	39	0	0.00%	100	0	0.00%
CDL/Non-Revenue Vehicle	26	0	0.00%	11	0	0.00%	21	0	0.00%
Armed Security Personnel	100	0	0.00%	0	0	0.00%	0	0	0.00%
RANDOM									
Revenue Vehicle Operations	21,705	21	0.10%	2,012	0	0.00%	4,037	4	0.10%
Vehicle and Equipment Maintenance	7,493	8	0.11%	398	1	0.25%	346	1	0.29%
Revenue Vehicle Control/Dispatch	1,926	3	0.16%	244	0	0.00%	540	1	0.19%
CDL/Non-Revenue Vehicle	1,269	2	0.16%	54	0	0.00%	129	1	0.78%
Armed Security Personnel	848	0	0.00%	1	0	0.00%	0	0	0.00%

Table 4-6. Alcohol Test Results by Test Type and Employee Category by Size (continued)

Employee Category	Large			Small			Rural		
	Number of Screening Tests	Number of Results ≥ 0.04	Percent ≥ 0.04	Number of Screening Tests	Number of Results ≥ 0.04	Percent ≥ 0.04	Number of Screening Tests	Number of Results ≥ 0.04	Percent ≥ 0.04
POST-ACCIDENT									
Revenue Vehicle Operations	11,136	3	0.03%	913	0	0.00%	682	1	0.15%
Vehicle and Equipment Maintenance	638	0	0.00%	73	0	0.00%	23	0	0.00%
Revenue Vehicle Control/Dispatch	134	0	0.00%	11	0	0.00%	9	0	0.00%
CDL/Non-Revenue Vehicle	86	1	1.16%	0	0	0.00%	10	0	0.00%
Armed Security Personnel	68	0	0.00%	0	0	0.00%	0	0	0.00%
REASONABLE SUSPICION									
Revenue Vehicle Operations	804	51	6.34%	32	7	21.88%	40	6	15.00%
Vehicle and Equipment Maintenance	115	10	8.70%	1	0	0.00%	5	1	20.00%
Revenue Vehicle Control/Dispatch	28	3	10.71%	0	0	0.00%	2	2	100.00%
CDL/Non-Revenue Vehicle	11	1	9.09%	1	0	0.00%	1	0	0.00%
Armed Security Personnel	2	0	0.00%	0	0	0.00%	0	0	0.00%
RETURN-TO-DUTY									
Revenue Vehicle Operations	390	0	0.00%	16	0	0.00%	11	0	0.00%
Vehicle and Equipment Maintenance	145	0	0.00%	1	0	0.00%	5	0	0.00%
Revenue Vehicle Control/Dispatch	17	0	0.00%	1	0	0.00%	0	0	0.00%
CDL/Non-Revenue Vehicle	11	0	0.00%	0	0	0.00%	0	0	0.00%
Armed Security Personnel	1	0	0.00%	0	0	0.00%	0	0	0.00%
FOLLOW-UP									
Revenue Vehicle Operations	3,702	9	0.24%	37	0	0.00%	46	0	0.00%
Vehicle and Equipment Maintenance	2,026	1	0.05%	26	0	0.00%	4	0	0.00%
Revenue Vehicle Control/Dispatch	310	0	0.00%	2	0	0.00%	0	0	0.00%
CDL/Non-Revenue Vehicle	300	0	0.00%	0	0	0.00%	0	0	0.00%
Armed Security Personnel	31	0	0.00%	0	0	0.00%	0	0	0.00%

Table 4-7. Alcohol Test Results by Employee Category and Test Type by Transit System and Contractor

Employee Category	Transit Systems			Contractors			Totals		
	Number of Screening Tests	Number of Results ≥ 0.04	Percent ≥ 0.04	Number of Screening Tests	Number of Results ≥ 0.04	Percent ≥ 0.04	Number of Screening Tests	Number of Results ≥ 0.04	Percent ≥ 0.04
TOTALS BY EMPLOYEE CATEGORY, ALL TEST TYPES									
Revenue Vehicle Operations	39,881	73	0.18%	10,819	31	0.29%	50,700	104	0.21%
Revenue Veh. and Equip. Maint.	10,252	17	0.17%	1,602	5	0.31%	11,854	22	0.19%
Revenue Veh. Control/Dispatch	2,714	7	0.26%	756	2	0.26%	3,470	9	0.26%
CDL / Non-Revenue Vehicle	1,872	5	0.27%	58	0	0.00%	1,930	5	0.26%
Armed Security Personnel	822	0	0.00%	229	0	0.00%	1,051	0	0.00%
TOTALS	55,541	102	0.18%	13,464	38	0.28%	69,005	140	0.20%

Test Type	Transit Systems			Contractors			Totals		
	Number of Screening Tests	Number of Results ≥ 0.04	Percent ≥ 0.04	Number of Screening Tests	Number of Results ≥ 0.04	Percent ≥ 0.04	Number of Screening Tests	Number of Results ≥ 0.04	Percent ≥ 0.04
REVENUE VEHICLE OPERATIONS									
Pre-Employment	3,107	2	0.06%	2,030	0	0.00%	5,137	2	0.04%
Random	22,039	19	0.09%	5,715	6	0.10%	27,754	25	0.09%
Post-Accident	10,239	4	0.04%	2,492	0	0.00%	12,731	4	0.03%
Reasonable Suspicion	659	40	6.07%	217	24	11.06%	876	64	7.31%
Return-to-Duty	380	0	0.00%	37	0	0.00%	417	0	0.00%
Follow-Up	3,457	8	0.23%	328	1	0.30%	3,785	9	0.24%
REVENUE VEHICLE AND EQUIPMENT MAINTENANCE									
Pre-Employment	389	0	0.00%	166	0	0.00%	555	0	0.00%
Random	7,052	7	0.10%	1,185	3	0.25%	8,237	10	0.12%
Post-Accident	638	0	0.00%	96	0	0.00%	734	0	0.00%
Reasonable Suspicion	112	9	8.04%	9	2	22.22%	121	11	9.09%
Return-to-Duty	138	0	0.00%	13	0	0.00%	151	0	0.00%
Follow-Up	1,923	1	0.05%	133	0	0.00%	2,056	1	0.05%

Table 4-7. Alcohol Test Results by Employee Category and Test Type by Transit System and Contractor (continued)

Test Type	Transit Systems			Contractors			Totals		
	Number of Screening Tests	Number of Results ≥ 0.04	Percent ≥ 0.04	Number of Screening Tests	Number of Results ≥ 0.04	Percent ≥ 0.04	Number of Screening Tests	Number of Results ≥ 0.04	Percent ≥ 0.04
REVENUE VEHICLE CONTROL/DISPATCH									
Pre-Employment	159	0	0.00%	87	0	0.00%	246	0	0.00%
Random	2,122	4	0.19%	588	0	0.00%	2,710	4	0.15%
Post-Accident	143	0	0.00%	11	0	0.00%	154	0	0.00%
Reasonable Suspicion	23	3	13.04%	7	2	28.57%	30	5	16.67%
Return-to-Duty	16	0	0.00%	2	0	0.00%	18	0	0.00%
Follow-Up	251	0	0.00%	61	0	0.00%	312	0	0.00%
CDL/NON-REVENUE VEHICLE									
Pre-Employment	57	0	0.00%	1	0	0.00%	58	0	0.00%
Random	1,399	3	0.21%	53	0	0.00%	1,452	3	0.21%
Post-Accident	92	1	1.09%	4	0	0.00%	96	1	1.04%
Reasonable Suspicion	13	1	7.69%	0	0	0.00%	13	1	7.69%
Return-to-Duty	11	0	0.00%	0	0	0.00%	11	0	0.00%
Follow-Up	300	0	0.00%	0	0	0.00%	300	0	0.00%
ARMED SECURITY PERSONNEL									
Pre-Employment	33	0	0.00%	67	0	0.00%	100	0	0.00%
Random	688	0	0.00%	161	0	0.00%	849	0	0.00%
Post-Accident	67	0	0.00%	1	0	0.00%	68	0	0.00%
Reasonable Suspicion	2	0	0.00%	0	0	0.00%	2	0	0.00%
Return-to-Duty	1	0	0.00%	0	0	0.00%	1	0	0.00%
Follow-Up	31	0	0.00%	0	0	0.00%	31	0	0.00%

Table 4-8. Alcohol Test Results by Employee Category and Test Type by Size

Employee Category	Large			Small			Rural		
	Number of Screening Tests	Number of Results ≥ 0.04	Percent ≥ 0.04	Number of Screening Tests	Number of Results ≥ 0.04	Percent ≥ 0.04	Number of Screening Tests	Number of Results ≥ 0.04	Percent ≥ 0.04
TOTALS BY EMPLOYEE CATEGORY, ALL TEST TYPES									
Revenue Vehicle Operations	41,119	85	0.21%	3,789	7	0.18%	5,792	12	0.21%
Revenue Veh. and Equip. Maint.	10,818	19	0.18%	614	1	0.16%	422	2	0.47%
Revenue Veh. Control / Dispatch	2,522	6	0.24%	297	0	0.00%	651	3	0.46%
CDL/Non-Revenue Vehicle	1,703	4	0.23%	66	0	0.00%	161	1	0.62%
Armed Security Personnel	1,050	0	0.00%	1	0	0.00%	0	0	0.00%
TOTALS	57,212	114	0.20%	4,769	8	0.17%	7,026	18	0.26%

Test Type	Large			Small			Rural		
	Number of Screening Tests	Number of Results ≥ 0.04	Percent ≥ 0.04	Number of Screening Tests	Number of Results ≥ 0.04	Percent ≥ 0.04	Number of Screening Tests	Number of Results ≥ 0.04	Percent ≥ 0.04
REVENUE VEHICLE OPERATIONS									
Pre-Employment	3,382	1	0.03%	779	0	0.00%	976	1	0.10%
Random	21,705	21	0.10%	2,012	0	0.00%	4,037	4	0.10%
Post-Accident	11,136	3	0.03%	913	0	0.00%	682	1	0.15%
Reasonable Suspicion	804	51	6.34%	32	7	21.88%	40	6	15.00%
Return-to-Duty	390	0	0.00%	16	0	0.00%	11	0	0.00%
Follow-Up	3,702	9	0.24%	37	0	0.00%	45	0	0.00%
REVENUE VEHICLE AND EQUIPMENT MAINTENANCE									
Pre-Employment	401	0	0.00%	115	0	0.00%	39	0	0.00%
Random	7,493	8	0.11%	398	1	0.25%	346	1	0.29%
Post-Accident	638	0	0.00%	73	0	0.00%	23	0	0.00%
Reasonable Suspicion	115	10	8.70%	1	0	0.00%	5	1	20.00%
Return-to-Duty	145	0	0.00%	1	0	0.00%	5	0	0.00%
Follow-Up	2,026	1	0.05%	26	0	0.00%	4	0	0.00%

Table 4-8. Alcohol Test Results by Employee Category and Test Type by Size (continued)

Test Type	Large			Small			Rural		
	Number of Screening Tests	Number of Results ≥ 0.04	Percent ≥ 0.04	Number of Screening Tests	Number of Results ≥ 0.04	Percent ≥ 0.04	Number of Screening Tests	Number of Results ≥ 0.04	Percent ≥ 0.04
REVENUE VEHICLE CONTROL/DISPATCH									
Pre-Employment	107	0	0.00%	39	0	0.00%	100	0	0.00%
Random	1,926	3	0.16%	244	0	0.00%	540	1	0.19%
Post-Accident	134	0	0.00%	11	0	0.00%	9	0	0.00%
Reasonable Suspicion	28	3	10.71%	0	0	0.00%	2	2	100.00%
Return-to-Duty	17	0	0.00%	1	0	0.00%	0	0	0.00%
Follow-Up	310	0	0.00%	2	0	0.00%	0	0	0.00%
CDL/NON-REVENUE VEHICLE									
Pre-Employment	26	0	0.00%	11	0	0.00%	21	0	0.00%
Random	1,269	2	0.16%	54	0	0.00%	129	1	0.78%
Post-Accident	86	1	1.16%	0	0	0.00%	10	0	0.00%
Reasonable Suspicion	11	1	9.09%	1	0	0.00%	1	0	0.00%
Return-to-Duty	11	0	0.00%	0	0	0.00%	0	0	0.00%
Follow-Up	300	0	0.00%	0	0	0.00%	0	0	0.00%
ARMED SECURITY PERSONNEL									
Pre-Employment	100	0	0.00%	0	0	0.00%	0	0	0.00%
Random	848	0	0.00%	1	0	0.00%	0	0	0.00%
Post-Accident	68	0	0.00%	0	0	0.00%	0	0	0.00%
Reasonable Suspicion	2	0	0.00%	0	0	0.00%	0	0	0.00%
Return-to-Duty	1	0	0.00%	0	0	0.00%	0	0	0.00%
Follow-Up	31	0	0.00%	0	0	0.00%	0	0	0.00%

4.3   Alcohol Testing Refusals

The FTA regulations stipulate that no employer shall permit an employee to perform safety-sensitive functions if the employee refuses a required alcohol test. The number of employees who refused to be tested was 51, as shown in Figure 4-4.

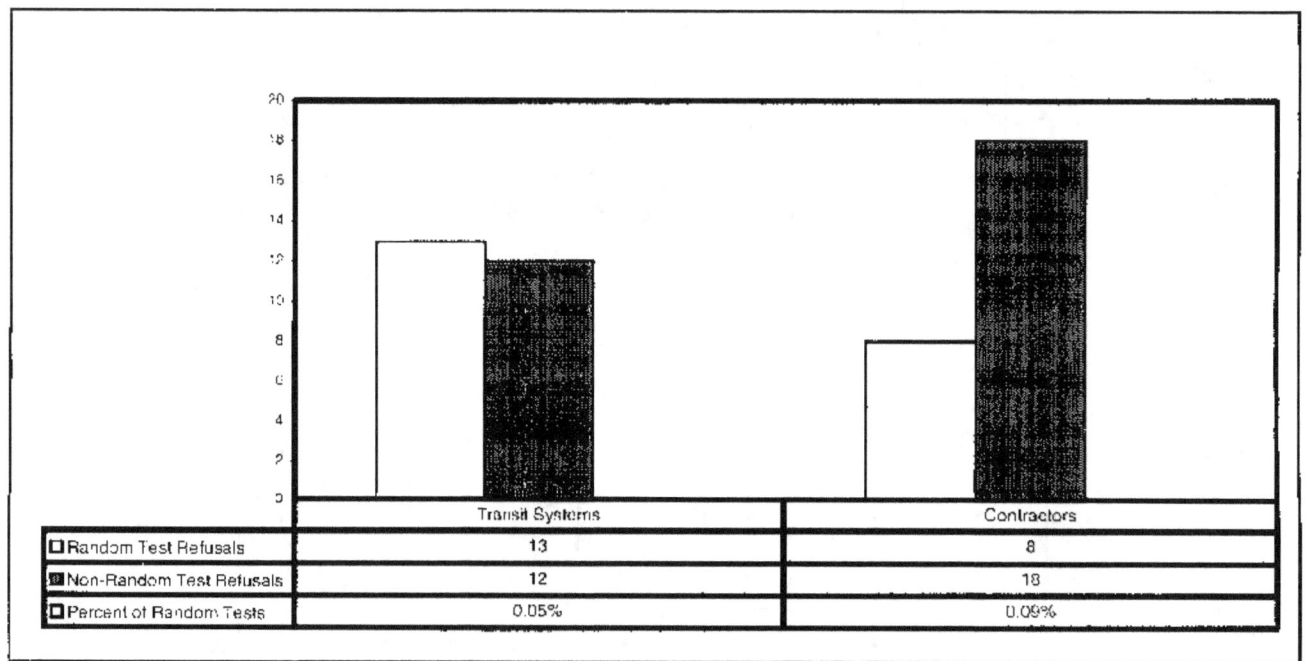

	Transit Systems	Contractors
☐ Random Test Refusals	13	8
▨ Non-Random Test Refusals	12	18
☐ Percent of Random Tests	0.05%	0.09%

Figure 4-4. Alcohol Test Refusals

4.4   Employees Returned to Duty

For 2000, 97 employees who had previously engaged in alcohol misuse or who had refused to take an alcohol test were returned to duty. Each individual had to undergo a return-to-duty test indicating a result of an alcohol concentration < 0.02. Table 4-9 shows the number of employees who returned-to-duty.

Table 4-9. Number of Covered Employees Who Returned-to-Duty

Employer	Returned-to-Duty	Percent of Total
Transit Systems	79	81.4%
Contractors	18	18.6%
Totals	97	100.0%

4.5 Accidents

FTA regulations require testing for drugs and alcohol following an accident in which there is a loss of human life. For non-fatal accidents meeting FTA-defined conditions, testing is required unless the covered employee's performance can be discounted completely as a causative or contributing factor. The definition of an accident can be found in Section 3.4.

Post-accident drug tests must be performed within 32 hours of an accident meeting the above-described conditions; **post-accident alcohol tests must be performed within 8 hours**. According to the regulations, employers should be conducting an equal number of drug and alcohol post-accident tests (i.e., with each accident requiring testing, both a drug and alcohol post-accident test should be performed). If both tests are not conducted, the reason should be documented.

Tables 4-10 and 4-11 present the 2000 accident data for non-fatal and fatal accidents with alcohol positives, by both transit systems and contractors and by size, respectively.

Table 4-10. Accidents with Alcohol Positives

Employer	Number of Non-Fatal Accidents	Number of Fatal Accidents	Number of Fatalities
Transit Systems	6	0	0
Contractors	0	0	0
Totals	6	0	0

Table 4-11. Accidents with Alcohol Positives by Size

Employer	Number of Non-Fatal Accidents	Number of Fatal Accidents	Number of Fatalities
Large	4	0	0
Small	1	0	0
Rural	1	0	0
Totals	6	0	0

4.6   Post-Accident Positives

Employers are required to report the number of accidents that result in a post-accident alcohol test indicating an alcohol concentration ≥ 0.04. The figures for 2000 are illustrated in Table 4-12 below.

Table 4-12. Post-Accident Alcohol Positives

Employer	Revenue Vehicle Operations	Vehicle and Equip. Maint.	Rev. Vehicle Cntl/Dsptch	CDL/Non-Revenue	Armed Security Personnel
Number 0.02 – 0.04	8	1	0	0	0
Number ≥ 0.04	4	0	0	1	0
Totals	12	1	0	1	0

4.7   Violation Rate

The FTA alcohol testing rule defines the violation rate as the number of random alcohol test results ≥ 0.04 plus the number of FTA-covered employees who refused a random test, divided by the total number of random tests plus the number of FTA-covered employees who refused a random test. See Tables 4-13 to 4-15 for data on violation rates for transit systems and contractors as well as by employer size. Figure 4-5 illustrates the violation rate by region. The following formula demonstrates how the violation rate is determined.

$$\frac{\textit{Random alcohol test results} \geq 0.04\% + \textit{number refused random testing}}{\textit{Total random tests} + \textit{number refused random testing}} = \frac{(42 + 21)}{(41,002 + 21)} = \frac{63}{41,023} = 0.15\%$$

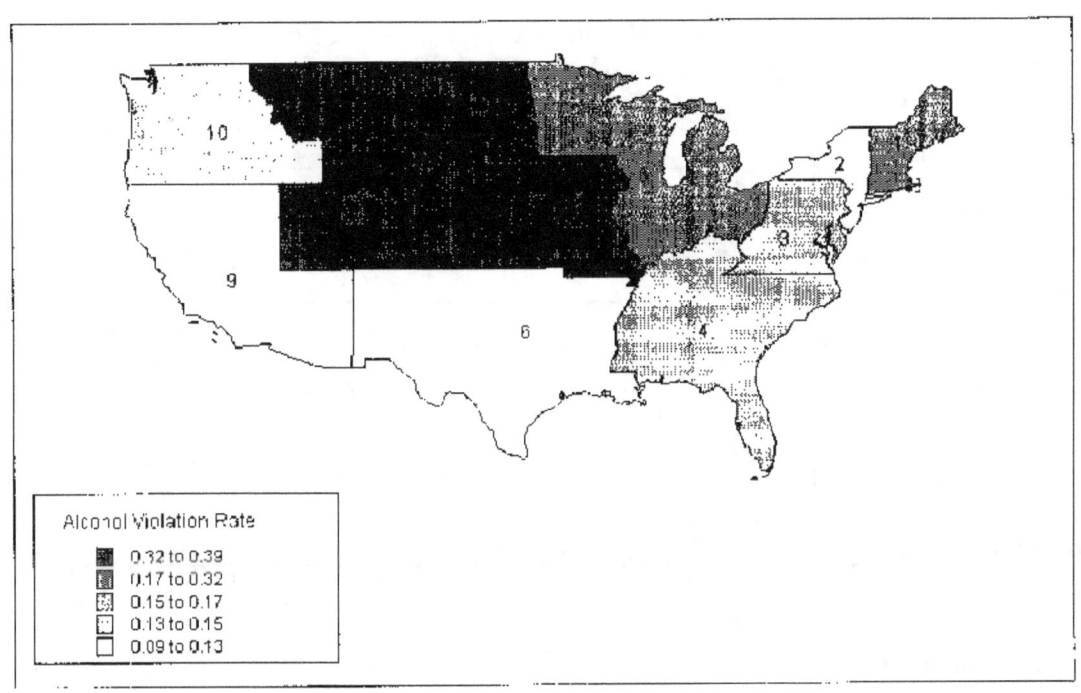

Figure 4-5. Alcohol Violation Rate by Region

Table 4-13. Violation Rate by Transit System/Contractor

Employer	Total Screens	Number ≥ 0.04	Random Test Refusals	Violation Rate
Transit Systems	33,300	33	13	0.14%
Contractors	7,702	9	8	0.23%
Totals	41,002	42	21	0.15%

Table 4-14. Violation Rate by Employer Size

Employer	Total Screens	Number ≥ 0.04	Random Test Refusals	Violation Rate
Large	33,241	34	13	0.11%
Small	2,709	1	3	0.15%
Rural	5,052	7	5	0.26%
Totals	41,002	42	21	0.15%

Table 4-15. Violation Rate by FTA Region

Region	Total Screens	Number ≥ 0.04	Random Test Refusals	Violation Rate
1	1,787	3	0	0.17%
2	8,448	8	4	0.14%
3	6,486	9	1	0.15%
4	6,470	3	7	0.15%
5	5,079	9	2	0.22%
6	4,550	3	1	0.09%
7	761	1	2	0.39%
8	937	2	1	0.32%
9	4,905	2	3	0.10%
10	1,579	2	0	0.13%
Totals	**41,002**	**42**	**21**	**0.15%**

4.8   Other Violations

Table 4-16 provides information for alcohol violations other than those detected through the alcohol testing process.

Table 4-16. Other Alcohol Violations

Number of Covered Employees	Transit Systems	Contractors	Other Violations
13	11	2	Covered employee used alcohol while performing safety-sensitive function.
13	12	1	Covered employee used alcohol within 4 hours of performing safety-sensitive function.
0	0	0	Covered employee used alcohol before taking a required post-accident alcohol test.
26	23	3	

5. TREND ANALYSIS

This chapter provides a trend analysis of the drug and alcohol testing conducted by all of the employers reporting in 1996, 1997, 1998, 1999, and 2000.

5.1   Drug and Alcohol Reports Received

In 1996, a total of 2,287 MIS forms were received and in 1997 there were 2,317 MIS forms submitted. In 1998, reporters could submit either hard copy MIS forms or data diskettes; the combined total of these in 1998 was 2,477. In 1999, there were 2,588 submissions, and in 2000 there were 2,657 submissions. Therefore, the number of drug and alcohol reports received has increased 16.2 percent over this 5-year period. The majority of this growth is due to the increased number of contractors reporting — this swell may be indicative of an industry-wide trend in contracting for services. Figure 5-1 illustrates this trend.

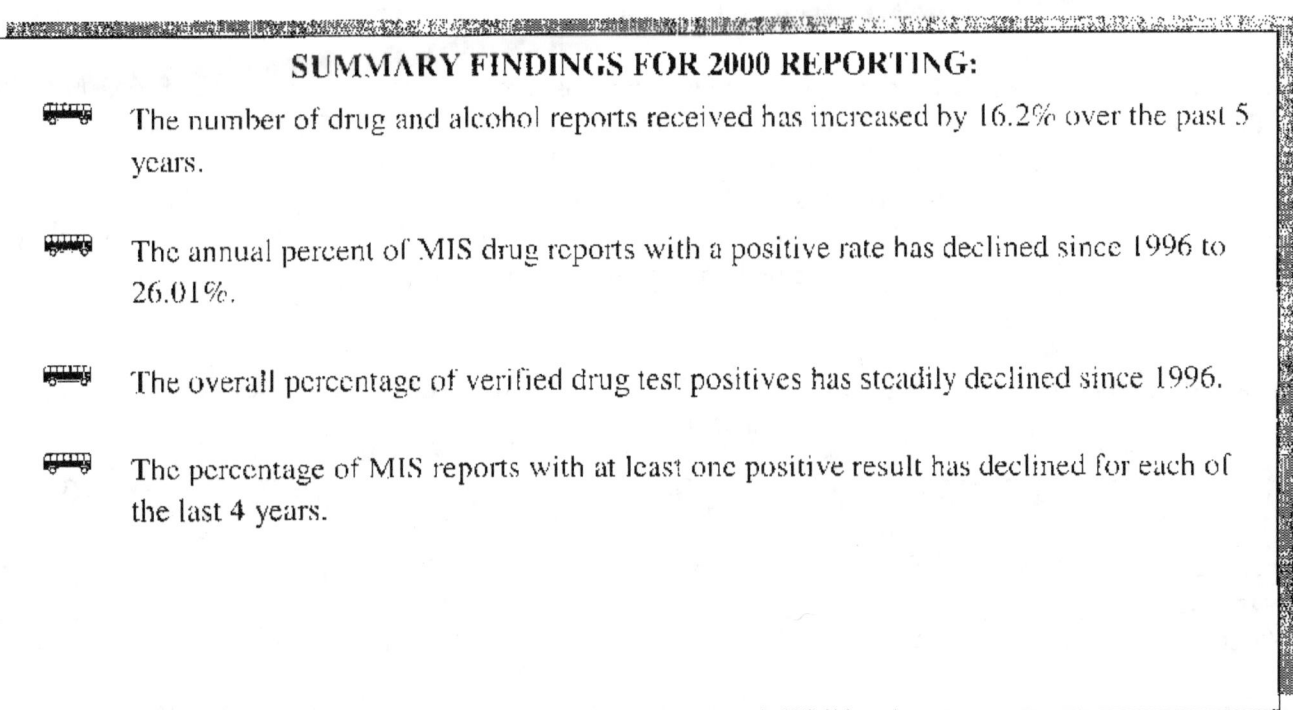

SUMMARY FINDINGS FOR 2000 REPORTING:

- The number of drug and alcohol reports received has increased by 16.2% over the past 5 years.

- The annual percent of MIS drug reports with a positive rate has declined since 1996 to 26.01%.

- The overall percentage of verified drug test positives has steadily declined since 1996.

- The percentage of MIS reports with at least one positive result has declined for each of the last 4 years.

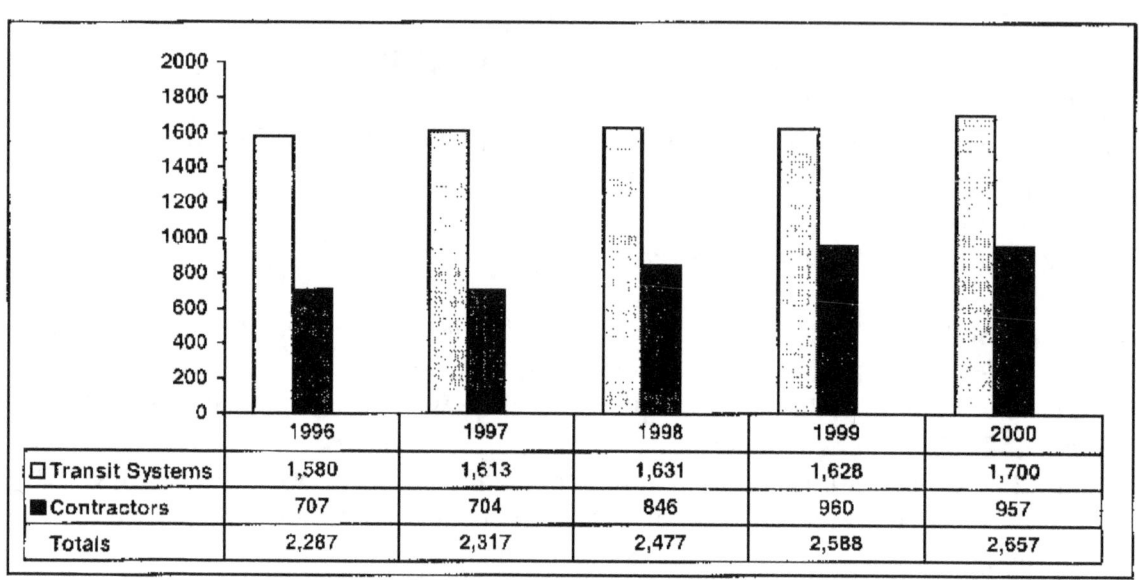

	1996	1997	1998	1999	2000
☐ Transit Systems	1,580	1,613	1,631	1,628	1,700
■ Contractors	707	704	846	960	957
Totals	2,287	2,317	2,477	2,588	2,657

Figure 5-1. Drug and Alcohol Reports Received

The total number of drug MIS reports with at least one positive test result has decreased for each of the last 5 years. For transit systems, the number increased slightly in 1999, after a steady decline from the preceding years, and it declined again in 2000. For contractors, their lowest rate of drug reports with positives was in 2000, although their rate was significantly higher than for transit systems for all 5 years. The total number of alcohol reports with test results ≥ 0.04 was on a downward trend with a slight increase in 2000, but with an overall decline in rates since 1996. See Table 5-1.

Table 5-1. Percent of Drug Reports with a Verified Positive and Alcohol Reports with a Test Result ≥ 0.04

Employer	Drug					Alcohol				
	1996	1997	1998	1999	2000	1996	1997	1998	1999	2000
Transit Systems	24.36	23.56	23.06	23.46	21.65	4.30	3.66	3.06	2.89	2.94
Contractors	37.34	40.91	35.10	33.96	33.75	3.82	4.26	5.08	2.40	3.24
Totals	**30.95**	**28.83**	**27.57**	**27.36**	**26.01**	**4.06**	**3.84**	**3.75**	**2.70**	**3.05**

5.2   Positive Drug and Alcohol Test Results

The transit industry-wide positive random drug test rate has declined over the last 5 years. Consistent with that trend is the random positive drug testing rate of the transit systems. Random alcohol test results ≥ 0.04 were in a downward trend until 2000, where the rate remained consistent with the previous year's rate. However, the results of contractor testing are not consistent with that trend. Contractors' positive random drug rates are at a much higher rate than transit systems and have fluctuated during the 5-year period. The overall rates for random positive drug test results have declined each year over the past 5 years with a downward trend experienced from 1996-1999, and a slight increase in 2000 for random alcohol test results ≥ 0.04. Table 5-2 shows the positive drug rate from 1996 to 2000. See Figures 5-2 and 5-3 for information on random drug and alcohol test results.

Table 5-2. Drug Positive Rate for 1996 to 2000

1996	1997	1998	1999	2000
1.60%	1.27%	1.20%	1.14%	1.05

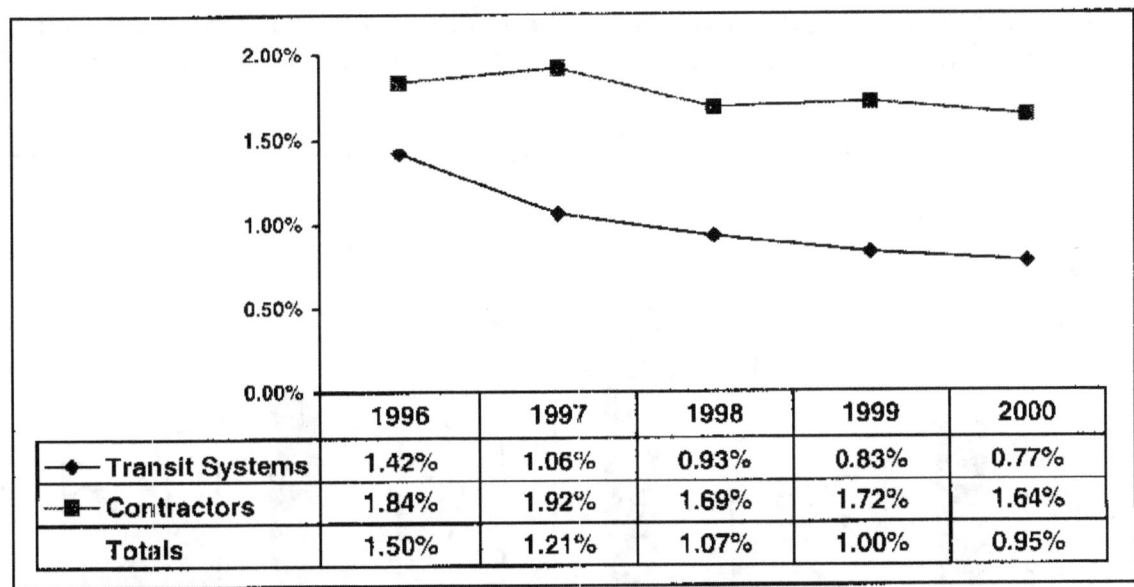

	1996	1997	1998	1999	2000
—◆— Transit Systems	1.42%	1.06%	0.93%	0.83%	0.77%
—■— Contractors	1.84%	1.92%	1.69%	1.72%	1.64%
Totals	1.50%	1.21%	1.07%	1.00%	0.95%

Figure 5-2. Comparison of Verified Positive Random Drug Test Results

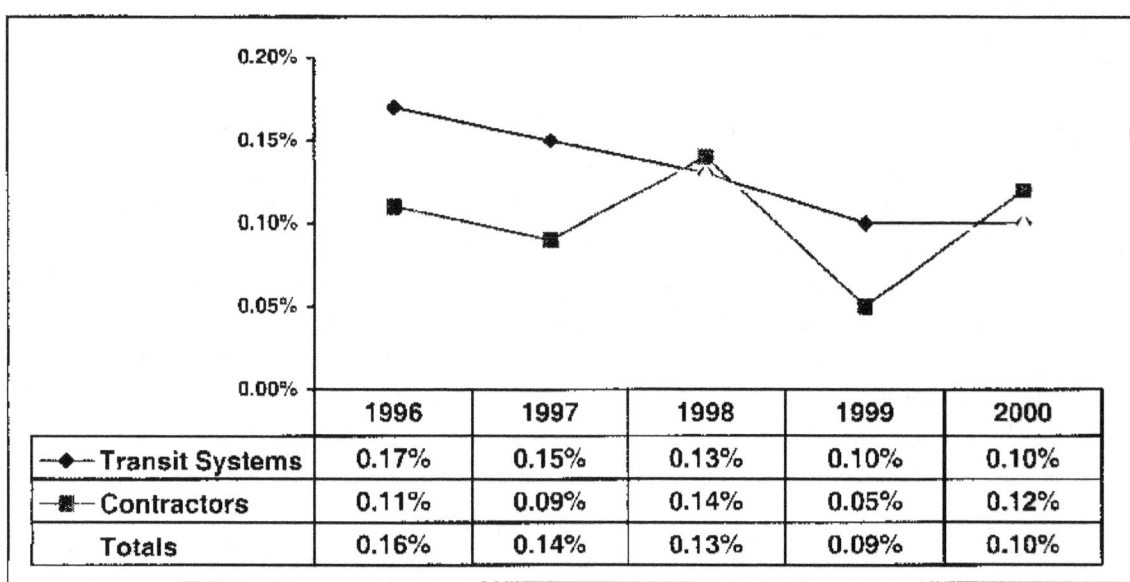

	1996	1997	1998	1999	2000
Transit Systems	0.17%	0.15%	0.13%	0.10%	0.10%
Contractors	0.11%	0.09%	0.14%	0.05%	0.12%
Totals	0.16%	0.14%	0.13%	0.09%	0.10%

Figure 5-3. Comparison of Random Alcohol Test Results ≥ 0.04

The positive drug test rate for all types of tests declined for the 1996-1999 time period, and has remained constant from 1999 to 2000. Test rates for contractors were substantially higher than those of transit systems. See Figure 5-4.

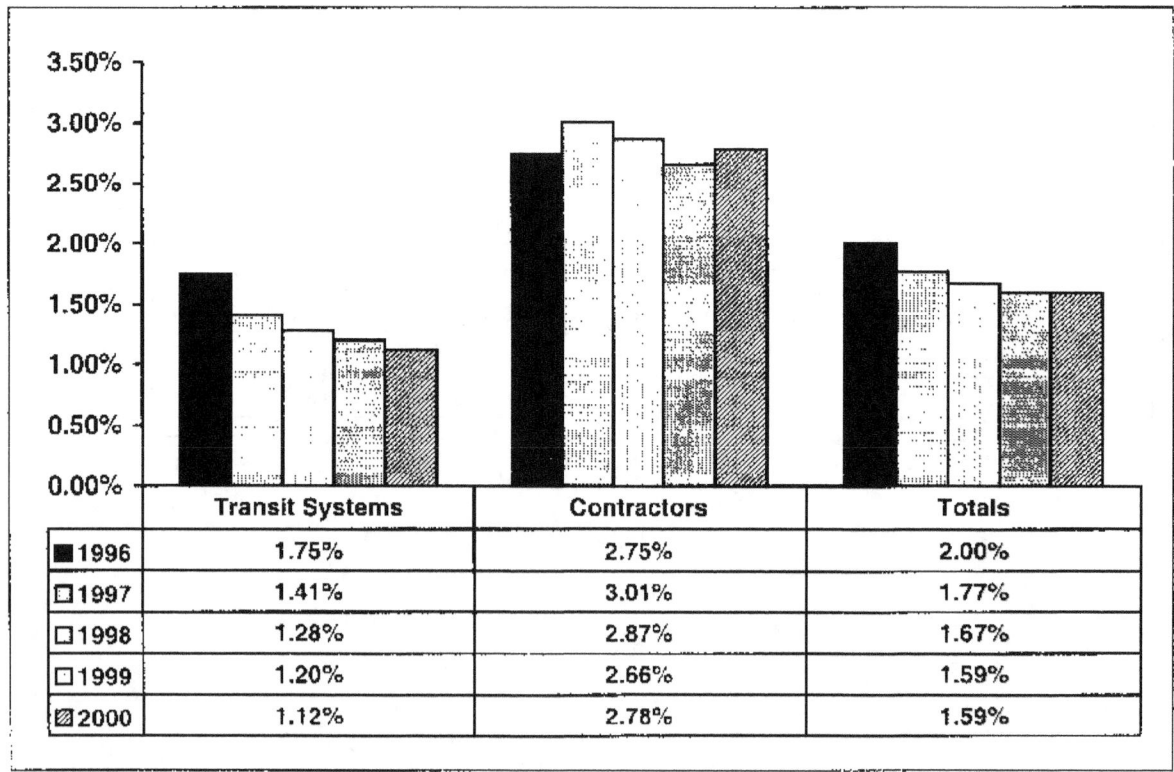

	Transit Systems	Contractors	Totals
1996	1.75%	2.75%	2.00%
1997	1.41%	3.01%	1.77%
1998	1.28%	2.87%	1.67%
1999	1.20%	2.66%	1.59%
2000	1.12%	2.78%	1.59%

Figure 5-4. Percent of Verified Drug Test Positives

The alcohol test rate ≥ 0.04 for all types of tests has remained fairly constant for 1996-1998, dipping slightly in 1999 and again in 2000, showing a downward trend from 1998 on. Test rates for contractors were higher than those of transit systems, particularly in 1998. See Figure 5-5.

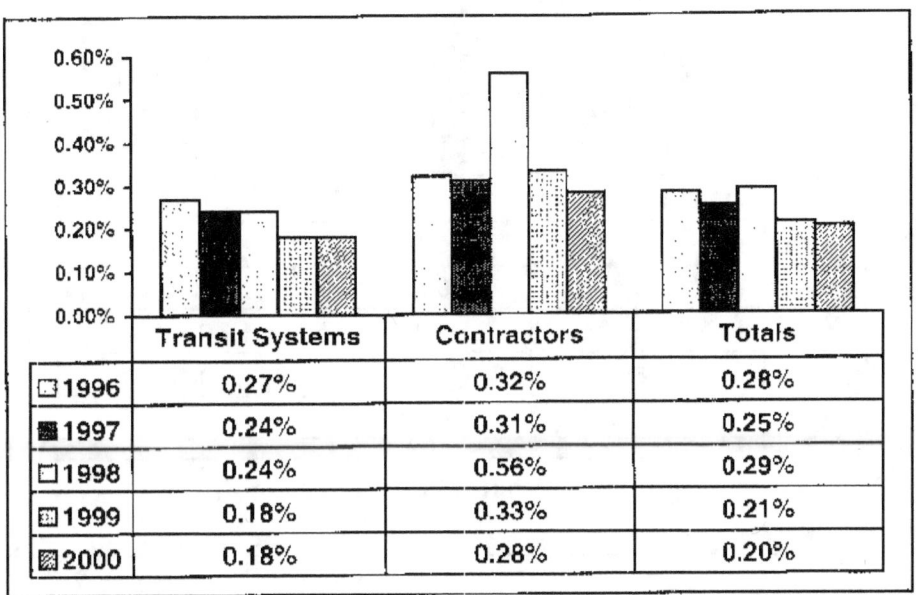

	Transit Systems	Contractors	Totals
☐ 1996	0.27%	0.32%	0.28%
■ 1997	0.24%	0.31%	0.25%
☐ 1998	0.24%	0.56%	0.29%
▦ 1999	0.18%	0.33%	0.21%
▨ 2000	0.18%	0.28%	0.20%

Figure 5-5. Percentage of All Alcohol Screening Test Results ≥ 0.04

5.3   Violation Rates and Test Refusals

See Figure 5-6 for the alcohol violation rate. In every year but 1996, contractors had a much greater violation rate than transit systems. In 1999, contractors nearly doubled transit systems in their violation rate. The overall trend has increased since 1996, and the total rate has fluctuated each year.

2000 Annual Report

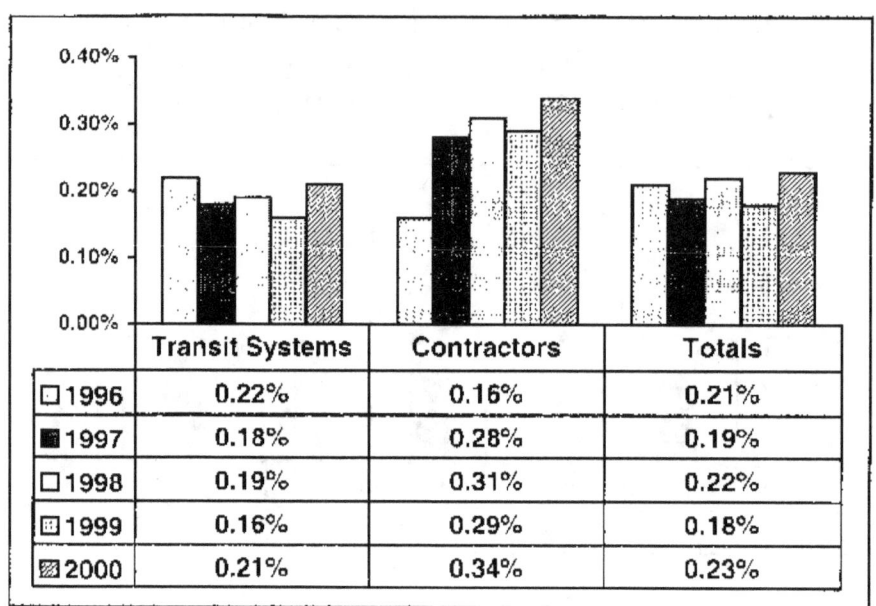

	Transit Systems	Contractors	Totals
□ 1996	0.22%	0.16%	0.21%
■ 1997	0.18%	0.28%	0.19%
□ 1998	0.19%	0.31%	0.22%
▦ 1999	0.16%	0.29%	0.18%
▨ 2000	0.21%	0.34%	0.23%

Figure 5-6. Violation Rate (Alcohol)

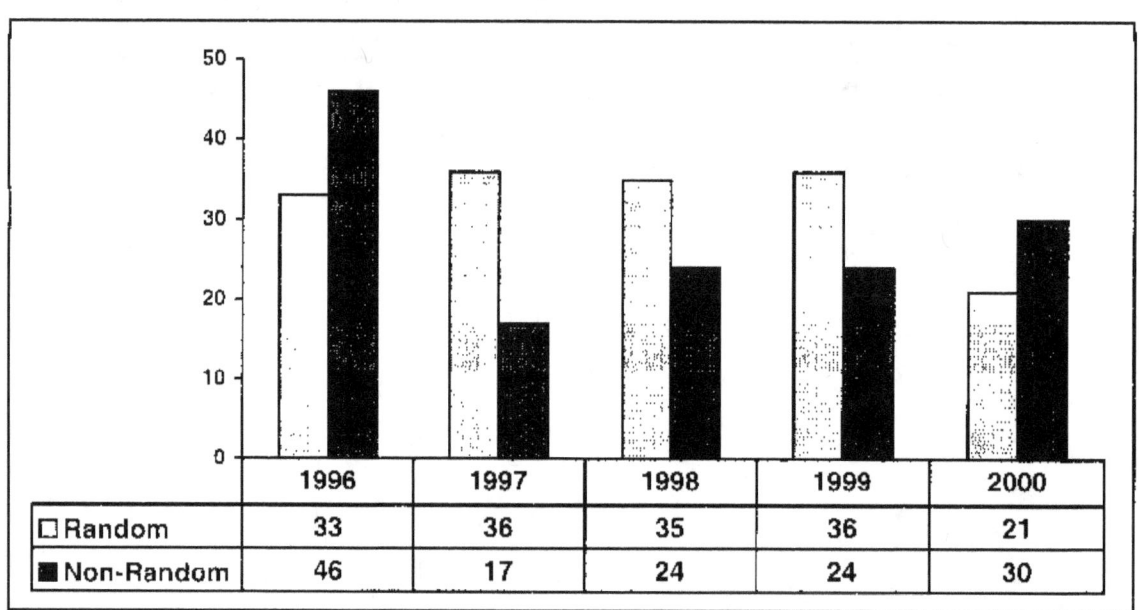

	1996	1997	1998	1999	2000
□ Random	33	36	35	36	21
■ Non-Random	46	17	24	24	30

Figure 5-7. Alcohol Test Refusals

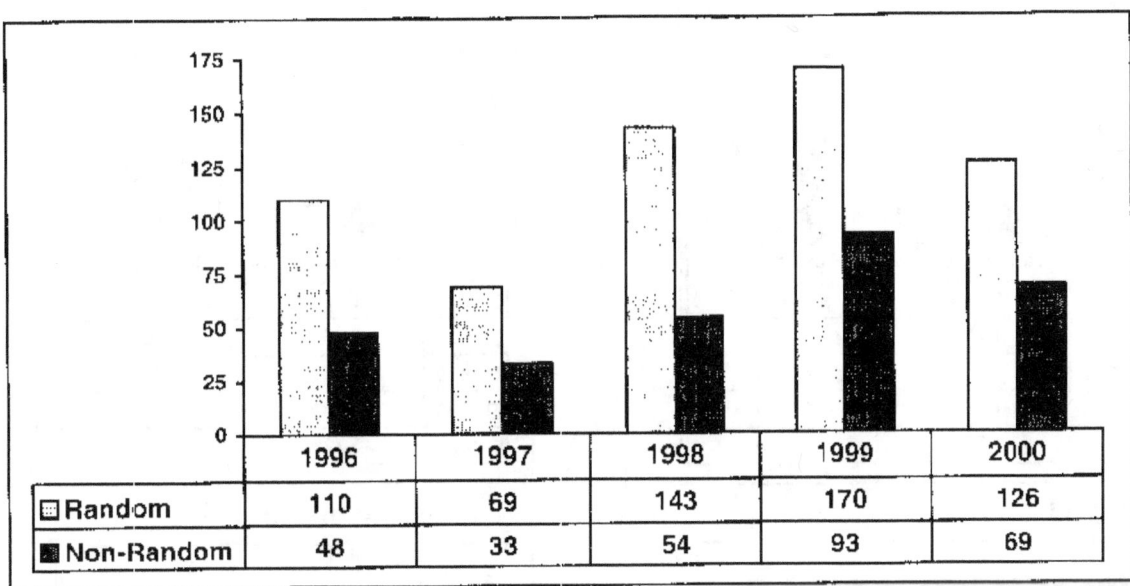

	1996	1997	1998	1999	2000
▦ Random	110	69	143	170	126
■ Non-Random	48	33	54	93	69

Figure 5-8. Drug Test Refusals

5.4   Drug and Alcohol Test Positives by Employment Category and Test Type

Figure 5-10 depicts the percent of verified drug test positives by test type for the last 5 years.

For return-to-duty testing, contractors had a greater percent of positives than in 1996, and an increase from the previous year. Post-accident positives for contractors also increased in 2000 from the previous year, as well as from the 1996 data.

All the testing categories for transit systems showed declines in the percent of positive tests in 2000, as compared to 1996. The testing categories for contractors of pre-employment, post-accident, and return-to-duty all showed increases in the percent positive in 2000 as compared to 1996. The testing categories of random, reasonable suspicion, and follow-up all showed declines in the percent positive in 2000 as compared to 1996.

The only testing category that showed a decline each year in positive test results was for random testing of transit systems.

For alcohol testing (see Figure 5-11), random positives for transit systems were the only test type that showed a decline in the percent of positive test results ≥ for each of the 4 years, with the fifth year being constant.

If comparing 1996 with 2000, there were less positives ≥ for both transit systems and contractors for post-accident and follow-up testing. Return-to-duty testing also showed a decline for transit systems and a constant percentage for contractors in comparison of the 1996 and 2000 data.

Pre-Employment

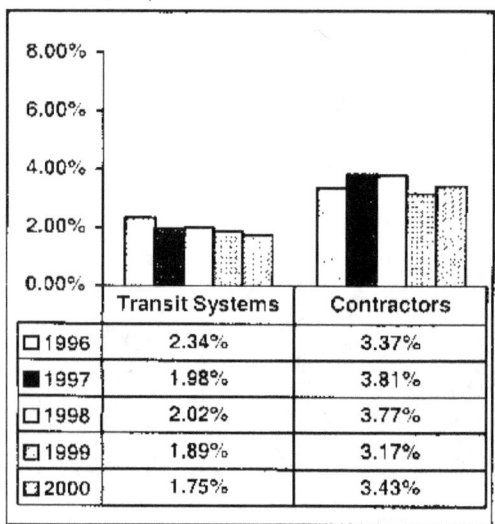

	Transit Systems	Contractors
☐ 1996	2.34%	3.37%
■ 1997	1.98%	3.81%
☐ 1998	2.02%	3.77%
⊞ 1999	1.89%	3.17%
▨ 2000	1.75%	3.43%

Random

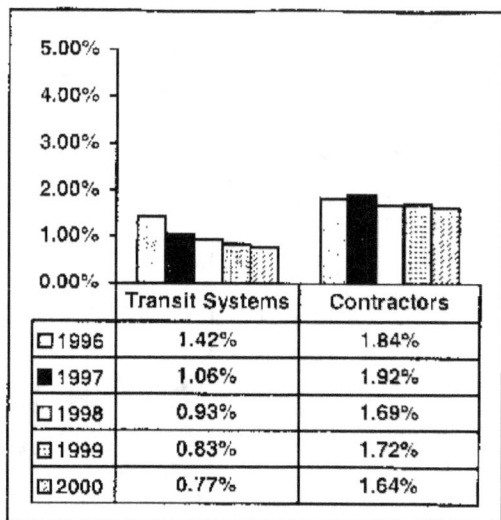

	Transit Systems	Contractors
☐ 1996	1.42%	1.84%
■ 1997	1.06%	1.92%
☐ 1998	0.93%	1.69%
⊞ 1999	0.83%	1.72%
▨ 2000	0.77%	1.64%

Post-Accident

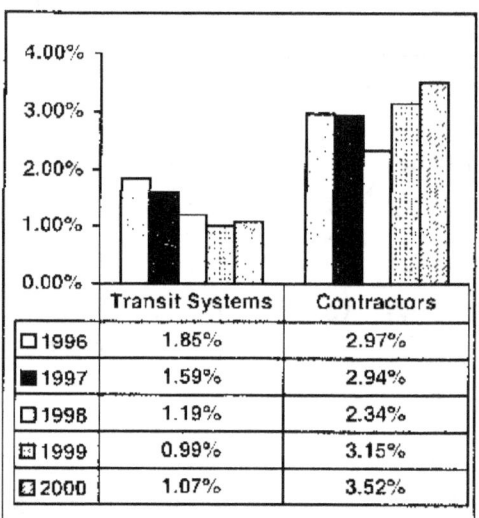

	Transit Systems	Contractors
☐ 1996	1.85%	2.97%
■ 1997	1.59%	2.94%
☐ 1998	1.19%	2.34%
⊞ 1999	0.99%	3.15%
▨ 2000	1.07%	3.52%

Reasonable Suspicion

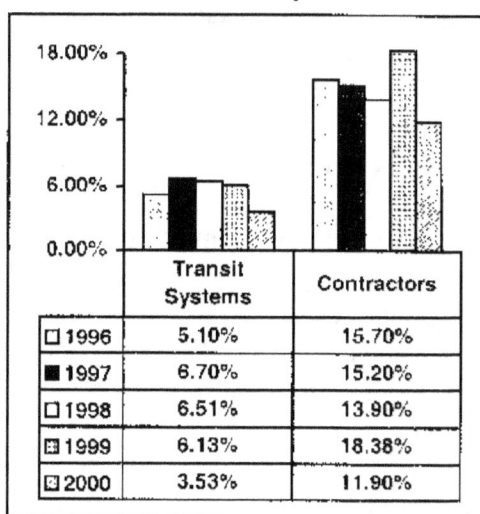

	Transit Systems	Contractors
☐ 1996	5.10%	15.70%
■ 1997	6.70%	15.20%
☐ 1998	6.51%	13.90%
⊞ 1999	6.13%	18.38%
▨ 2000	3.53%	11.90%

Return-to-Duty

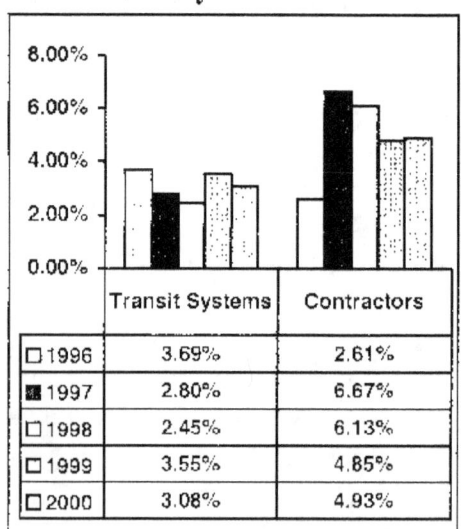

	Transit Systems	Contractors
☐ 1996	3.69%	2.61%
■ 1997	2.80%	6.67%
☐ 1998	2.45%	6.13%
⊞ 1999	3.55%	4.85%
☐ 2000	3.08%	4.93%

Follow-up

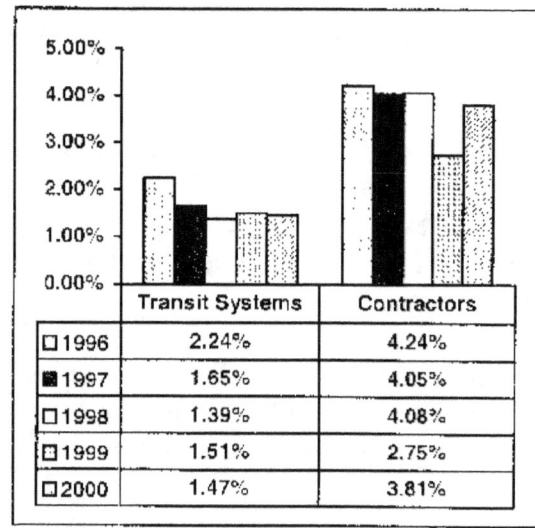

	Transit Systems	Contractors
☐ 1996	2.24%	4.24%
■ 1997	1.65%	4.05%
☐ 1998	1.39%	4.08%
⊞ 1999	1.51%	2.75%
☐ 2000	1.47%	3.81%

Figure 5-9. Drug Test Results by Test Type, 1996 to 2000

Post-Accident

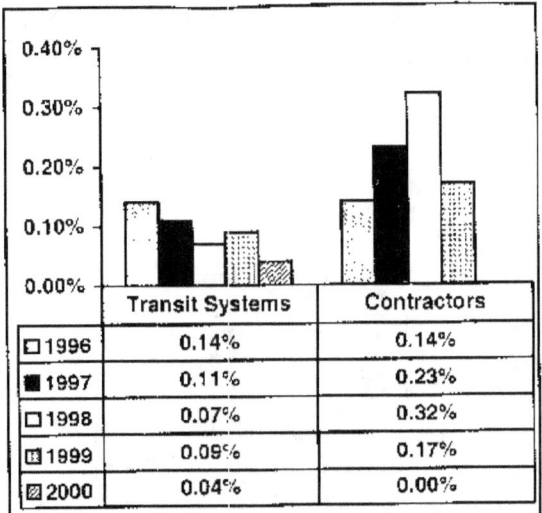

	Transit Systems	Contractors
☐ 1996	0.14%	0.14%
■ 1997	0.11%	0.23%
☐ 1998	0.07%	0.32%
⊞ 1999	0.09%	0.17%
▨ 2000	0.04%	0.00%

Reasonable Suspicion

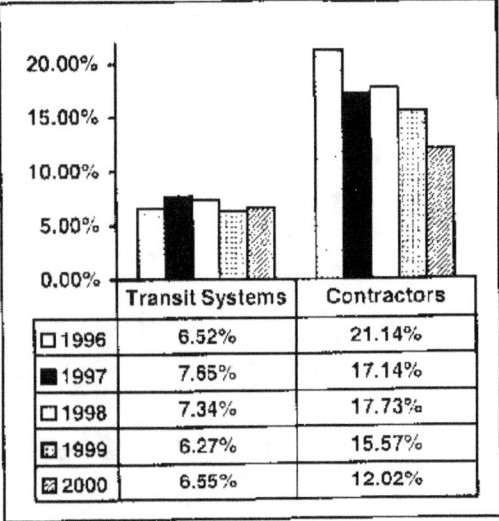

	Transit Systems	Contractors
☐ 1996	6.52%	21.14%
■ 1997	7.65%	17.14%
☐ 1998	7.34%	17.73%
⊞ 1999	6.27%	15.57%
▨ 2000	6.55%	12.02%

Return-to-Duty

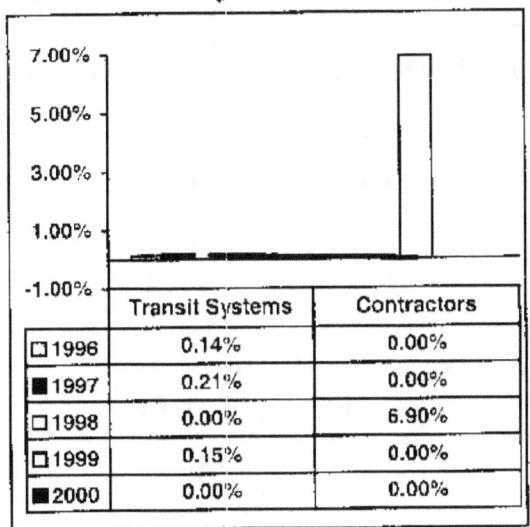

	Transit Systems	Contractors
☐ 1996	0.14%	0.00%
■ 1997	0.21%	0.00%
☐ 1998	0.00%	6.90%
☐ 1999	0.15%	0.00%
■ 2000	0.00%	0.00%

Follow-up

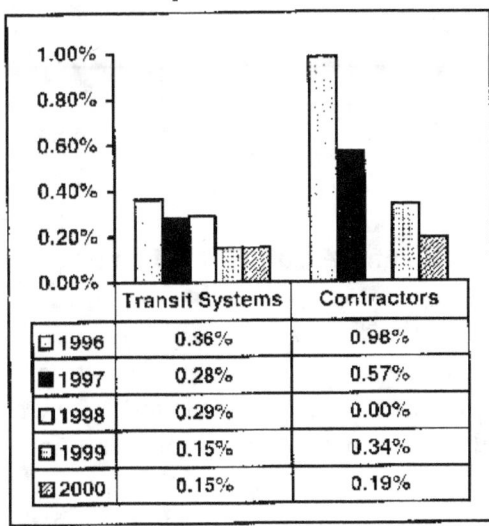

	Transit Systems	Contractors
☐ 1996	0.36%	0.98%
■ 1997	0.28%	0.57%
☐ 1998	0.29%	0.00%
⊞ 1999	0.15%	0.34%
▨ 2000	0.15%	0.19%

Random

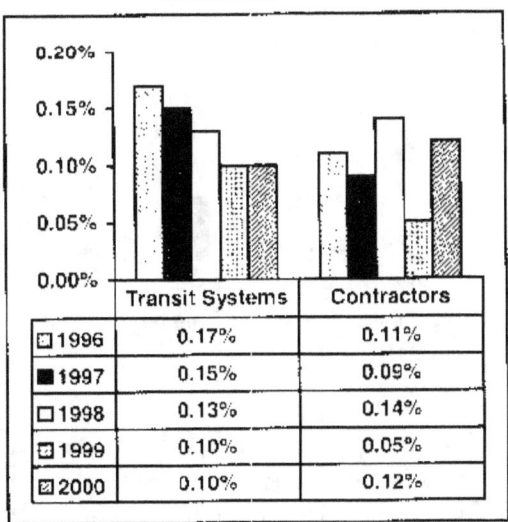

	Transit Systems	Contractors
☐ 1996	0.17%	0.11%
■ 1997	0.15%	0.09%
☐ 1998	0.13%	0.14%
⊞ 1999	0.10%	0.05%
▨ 2000	0.10%	0.12%

Figure 5-10. Alcohol Test Results ≥ 0.04 by Test Type, 1996 to 2000

Figure 5-12 compares test results by drug type from 1996 to 2000. As shown, marijuana (THC) was the predominant drug found in pre-employment, random, and post-accident testing. Cocaine was the most frequently detected drug in the reasonable suspicion, return-to-duty, and follow-up testing categories.

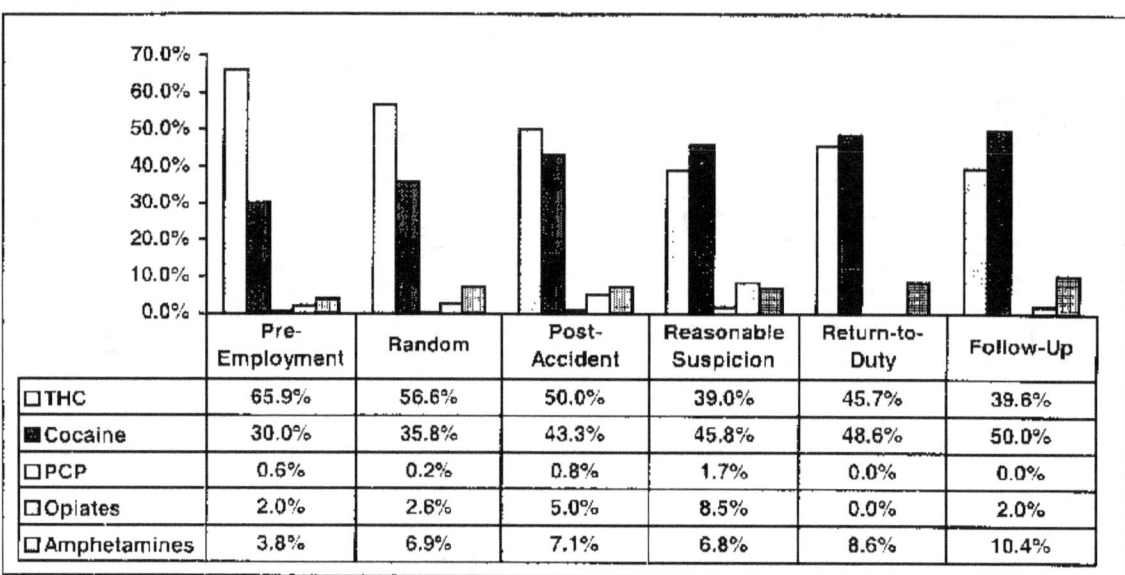

	Pre-Employment	Random	Post-Accident	Reasonable Suspicion	Return-to-Duty	Follow-Up
☐ THC	65.9%	56.6%	50.0%	39.0%	45.7%	39.6%
■ Cocaine	30.0%	35.8%	43.3%	45.8%	48.6%	50.0%
☐ PCP	0.6%	0.2%	0.8%	1.7%	0.0%	0.0%
☐ Opiates	2.0%	2.6%	5.0%	8.5%	0.0%	2.0%
☐ Amphetamines	3.8%	6.9%	7.1%	6.8%	8.6%	10.4%

Figure 5-11. Comparison of Verified Test Positives by Drug Type, 1996 to 2000

5.5 Drug and Alcohol Test Positives – Regional Comparisons

Figures 5-13 and 5-14 show random alcohol tests ≥ 0.04 and positive random drug test by region. Figure 5-15 depicts the percent of positive random drug tests by region. As shown, for each of the 5 years, marijuana was detected most frequently in positive samples, followed by cocaine. Amphetamines were the third most frequently detected, although in substantially smaller numbers; the highest percent of amphetamine positives was in 2000 with 5.39 percent. Specific percentages are cited in the following tables.

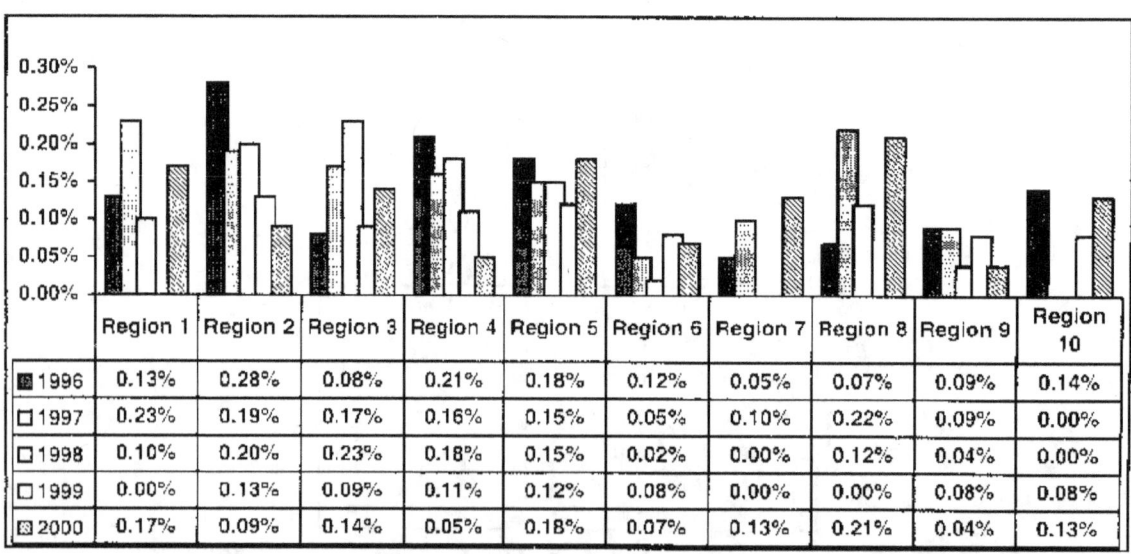

	Region 1	Region 2	Region 3	Region 4	Region 5	Region 6	Region 7	Region 8	Region 9	Region 10
■ 1996	0.13%	0.28%	0.08%	0.21%	0.18%	0.12%	0.05%	0.07%	0.09%	0.14%
☐ 1997	0.23%	0.19%	0.17%	0.16%	0.15%	0.05%	0.10%	0.22%	0.09%	0.00%
☐ 1998	0.10%	0.20%	0.23%	0.18%	0.15%	0.02%	0.00%	0.12%	0.04%	0.00%
☐ 1999	0.00%	0.13%	0.09%	0.11%	0.12%	0.08%	0.00%	0.00%	0.08%	0.08%
▦ 2000	0.17%	0.09%	0.14%	0.05%	0.18%	0.07%	0.13%	0.21%	0.04%	0.13%

Figure 5-12. Random Alcohol Test Results ≥ 0.04 by Region

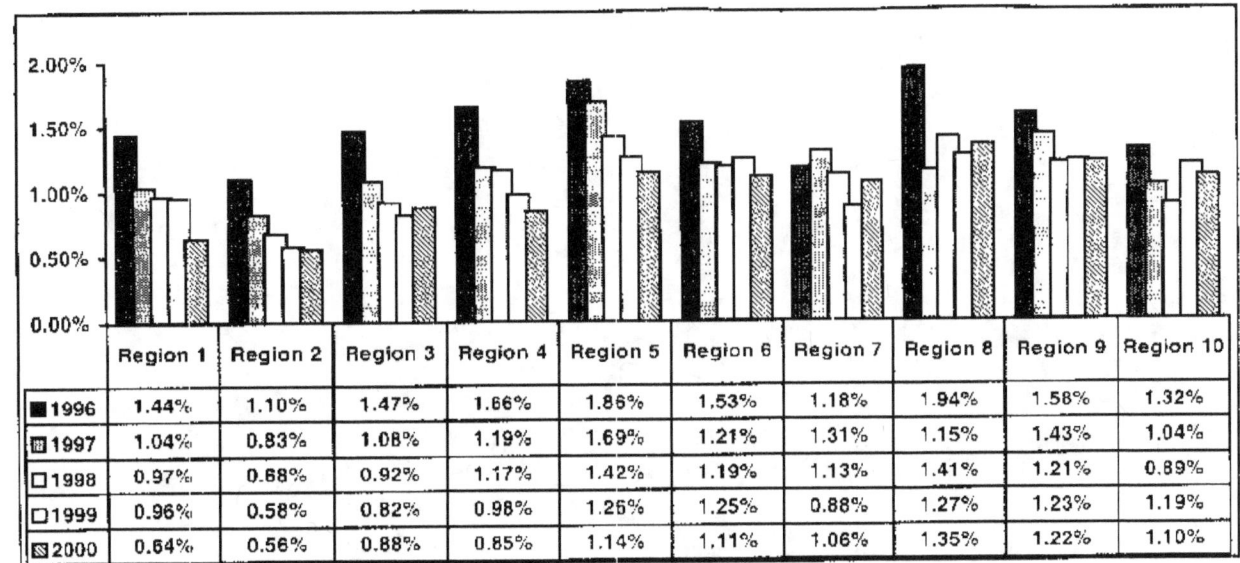

	Region 1	Region 2	Region 3	Region 4	Region 5	Region 6	Region 7	Region 8	Region 9	Region 10
■ 1996	1.44%	1.10%	1.47%	1.66%	1.86%	1.53%	1.18%	1.94%	1.58%	1.32%
▥ 1997	1.04%	0.83%	1.08%	1.19%	1.69%	1.21%	1.31%	1.15%	1.43%	1.04%
☐ 1998	0.97%	0.68%	0.92%	1.17%	1.42%	1.19%	1.13%	1.41%	1.21%	0.89%
☐ 1999	0.96%	0.58%	0.82%	0.98%	1.25%	1.25%	0.88%	1.27%	1.23%	1.19%
▨ 2000	0.64%	0.56%	0.88%	0.85%	1.14%	1.11%	1.06%	1.35%	1.22%	1.10%

Figure 5-13. Verified Positive Random Drug Tests by Region

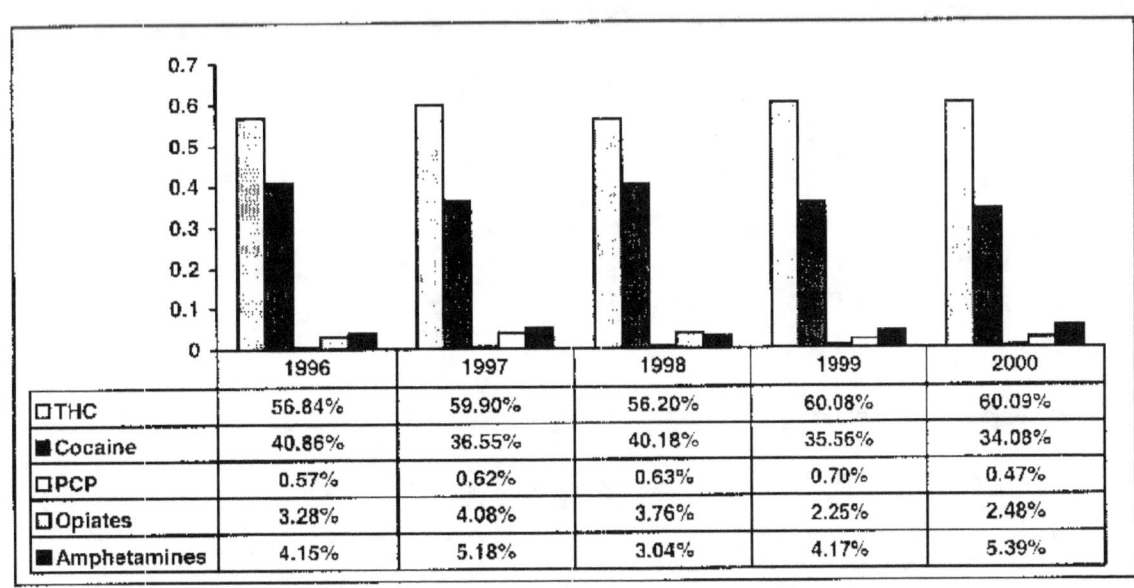

	1996	1997	1998	1999	2000
☐ THC	56.84%	59.90%	56.20%	60.08%	60.09%
■ Cocaine	40.86%	36.55%	40.18%	35.56%	34.08%
☐ PCP	0.57%	0.62%	0.63%	0.70%	0.47%
☐ Opiates	3.28%	4.08%	3.76%	2.25%	2.48%
■ Amphetamines	4.15%	5.18%	3.04%	4.17%	5.39%

Figure 5-14. Percent of Verified Positive Random Drug Tests by Drug Type

APPENDIX A

GLOSSARY

GLOSSARY

Accident: An occurrence associated with the operation of a vehicle, if as a result:
(1) An individual dies;
(2) An individual suffers a bodily injury and immediately receives medical treatment away from the scene of the accident;
(3) With respect to an occurrence in which the mass transit vehicle involved is a bus, electric bus, van, or automobile, one or more vehicles incurs disabling damage as the result of the occurrence and is transported away from the scene by a tow truck or other vehicle; or
(4) With respect to an occurrence in which the mass transit vehicle involved is a rail car, trolley car, trolley bus, or vessel, the mass transit vehicle is removed from revenue service.

Alcohol: The intoxicating agent in beverage alcohol, ethyl alcohol, or other low molecular weight alcohols including methyl or isopropyl alcohol.

Alcohol Concentration: The alcohol in a volume of breath expressed in terms of grams of alcohol per 210 liters of breath as indicated by a breath test.

Alcohol Use: The consumption of any beverage, mixture or preparation, including any medication containing alcohol.

Anti-Drug Program: A program to detect and deter the use of prohibited drugs as required by FTA regulations.

Armed Security Personnel: Function including any person who provides security to protect persons or property, and any person who carries a firearm.

Canceled or Invalid Test: In drug testing, a drug test that has been declared invalid by a Medical Review Officer (MRO). In alcohol testing, this would be a test that is deemed to be invalid. It is neither a positive nor a negative test.

CDL/Non-Revenue Vehicle: Job category including any transit employee who holds a Commercial Driver's License (CDL), performs a function requiring a CDL, and is not included in any other job category.

Confirmation (or Confirmatory) Test: In drug testing, a second analytical procedure to identify the presence of a specific drug or metabolite that is independent of the screening test and uses a different technique and chemical principle from that of the screening test in order to ensure reliability and accuracy. In alcohol testing, a second test following a screening test with a result of 0.02 or greater that provides quantitative data of alcohol concentration.

Consortium: An entity, including a group or association of employers, operators, recipients, subrecipients, or contractors, which provides drug testing services and acts on behalf of the employer.

Contractor: A person or organization that provides a service for a recipient, subrecipient, employer, or operator consistent with a specific understanding or arrangement. The understanding can be a written contract or an informal arrangement that reflects an ongoing relationship between the parties.

Covered Employee: A person, including an applicant, transferee, and certain volunteers who perform a safety-sensitive function for a recipient, subrecipient, employer, or operator.

DOT: Department of Transportation.

DOT Agency: An agency (or "operating administration") of the United States Department of Transportation administering regulations requiring drug testing.

Drug Metabolite: The specific substance produced when the human body metabolizes a given prohibited drug as it passes through the body and is excreted in urine.

Drug Test: The laboratory analysis of a urine specimen collected in accordance with 49 CFR Part 40 and analyzed in a DHHS-approved laboratory.

Education: Efforts that include the display and distribution of informational materials, a community service hotline telephone number for employee assistance, and the transit entity policy regarding drug use and alcohol misuse in the workplace.

Employee: An individual designated in a DOT agency regulation as subject to drug testing and/or alcohol testing. "Employee" includes an applicant for employment.

Employer: A recipient or other entity that provides mass transportation services or performs a safety-sensitive function for such recipient or other entity. This term includes subrecipients, operators, and contractors.

Follow-up Test: Required of employees who have returned to duty in a safety-sensitive position following a positive drug test result or an alcohol test result of ≥ 0.04. A minimum of six tests must be performed during the first 12 months after the employee returns-to-duty.

FTA: The Federal Transit Administration, an agency of the U.S. Department of Transportation.

Large Operator: A recipient or subrecipient primarily operating in an area of 200,000 or more in population.

Medical Review Officer (MRO): A licensed physician (Doctor of Medicine or Doctor of Osteopathy) responsible for receiving laboratory results generated by an employer's drug testing program, who has knowledge of substance abuse disorders and has appropriate medical training to interpret and evaluate an individual's confirmed positive test result together with appropriate medical history and any other relevant biomedical information.

Post-Accident Testing: Required testing for prohibited drugs and alcohol, following certain mass transit accidents. These accidents include those in which a death occurs, medical treatment away from the scene is required, or one or more of the vehicles involved incurs disabling damage.

Pre-Employment Testing: Testing that is designed to identify applicants who have consumed a prohibited drug in the recent past. Employers are prohibited from hiring an applicant for a safety-sensitive function unless they have a verified negative drug test.

Prohibited Drugs: Include marijuana (THC), cocaine, phencyclidine (PCP), opiates, and amphetamines.

Rail Operators: A recipient and its contractors and subrecipients that operate rapid transit operations within an urban area and are not connected to the general railroad system. Rail vehicles include railcars, trolley cars, and trolley buses.

Random Testing: Identifies employees who are using drugs or misusing alcohol by using an unpredictable and unannounced testing pattern.

Random Testing Rate: The number of drug tests equal to at least 50 percent of the total number of safety-sensitive employees, and alcohol tests equal to at least 10 percent of the total number of safety-sensitive employees must be conducted each year by this method.

Reasonable Suspicion Testing: Required when an employer has reasonable suspicion that an employee has used a prohibited drug or has misused alcohol as defined in the regulations. Reasonable suspicion testing must be based on specific, contemporaneous, articulable observations made by a trained supervisor concerning the appearance, behavior, speech, or body odor of a safety-sensitive employee.

Recipient: An entity receiving federal financial assistance under Section 5307, 5309, or 5311 of the Federal Transit Act or under sections 103(e)(4) of Title 23 of the U.S. Code.

Refuse to Submit (to an alcohol test): A covered employee fails to provide adequate breath for testing without a valid medical explanation.

Refuse to Submit (to a drug test): A covered employee fails to provide a urine sample as required by 49 CFR Part 40, without a valid medical explanation, after the employee has received notice of the requirement to be tested or engages in conduct that clearly obstructs the testing process.

Return-to-Duty Testing: Required before an employee is allowed to return to duty to perform a safety-sensitive function following a verified positive drug test, an alcohol result of 0.04 or greater, a refusal to submit to a test, or any other violation of the regulation.

Revenue Vehicle Control/Dispatch: Job function including any person who controls the dispatch or movement of revenue service vehicles.

Revenue Vehicle Operations: Function including any person who operates or works as a crewman on revenue service vehicles at any time.

Rural Operators: A subrecipient of 5311 funding primarily operating in an area of less than 50,000 in population.

Safety-Sensitive Function: Any of the following duties:

- Operating a revenue service vehicle, including when not in revenue service;
- Operating a non-revenue service vehicle, when required to be operated by a holder of a Commercial Driver's License;
- Controlling dispatch or movement of a revenue service vehicle;
- Maintaining a revenue service vehicle or equipment used in revenue service, unless the recipient receives section 5311 funding and contracts out such services; and/or
- Providing security and carrying a firearm.

Screening Test (or Initial Test): In drug testing, an immunoassay screen to eliminate "negative" urine specimens from further analysis. In alcohol testing, an analytic procedure to determine whether an employee may have a prohibited concentration of alcohol in a breath specimen.

Small Operators: A recipient or subrecipient primarily operating in an area equal to or greater than 50,000 and less than 200,000 in population.

Substance Abuse Professional (SAP): A licensed physician (Doctor of Medicine or Doctor of Osteopathy), or a licensed or certified psychologist, social worker, employee assistance professional, or addiction counselor (certified by the National Association of Alcoholism and Drug Abuse Counselors Certification Commission), with knowledge of and clinical experience in the diagnosis and treatment of drug and alcohol-related disorders.

Transit System: The public entity that receives the Federal grant (direct grant recipient), whether or not that recipient provides mass transit services directly.

Vehicle and Equipment Maintenance: Function including any person repairing or maintaining revenue service vehicles or other equipment used in revenue service.

Verified Negative (drug test result): A drug test result reviewed by a MRO and determined to have no evidence of prohibited drug use.

Verified Positive (drug test result): A drug test result reviewed by a MRO and determined to have evidence of prohibited drug use.

APPENDIX B

FTA REGIONS

The Federal Transit Administration is comprised of 10 regions, which are identified below. The data provided by these regions have facilitated the comparison of drug and alcohol test results and the identification of regional trends.

U.S. States and Territories Reporting to the 10 FTA Regions

Region 1	Region 2	Region 3	Region 4	Region 5
Connecticut	New Jersey	Delaware	Alabama	Illinois
Maine	New York	District of	Florida	Indiana
Massachusetts	Puerto Rico	Columbia	Georgia	Michigan
New Hampshire	Virgin Islands	Maryland	Kentucky	Minnesota
Rhode Island		Pennsylvania	Mississippi	Ohio
Vermont		Virginia	North Carolina	Wisconsin
		West Virginia	South Carolina	
			Tennessee	

Region 6	Region 7	Region 8	Region 9	Region 10
Arkansas	Iowa	Colorado	American Samoa	Alaska
Louisiana	Kansas	Montana	Arizona	Idaho
New Mexico	Missouri	North Dakota	California	Oregon
Oklahoma	Nebraska	South Dakota	Guam	Washington
Texas		Utah	Hawaii	
		Wyoming	Nevada	
			Northern	
			Mariana Islands	

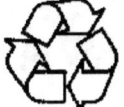